Is This Change Real?

Interpreting Patient Outcomes in
Physical Therapy

Daniel L. Riddle, PT, PhD, FAPTA
  Otto D. Payton Professor
  Department of Physical Therapy
  Virginia Commonwealth University
  Richmond, Virginia

Paul W. Stratford, PT, MSc
  Professor, School of Rehabilitation Science
  Associate Member
  Department of Clinical Epidemiology and Biostatistics
  McMaster University
  Hamilton, Ontario

 F.A. Davis Company • Philadelphia

F. A. Davis Company
1915 Arch Street
Philadelphia, PA 19103
www.fadavis.com

Printed in the United States of America

Last digit indicates print number: 10 9 8 7 6 5 4 3 2

Acquisitions Editor: Melissa Duffield
Manager of Content Development: George W. Lang
Developmental Editor: Lisa Consoli
Art and Design Manager: Carolyn O'Brien

As new scientific information becomes available through basic and clinical research, recommended treatments and drug therapies undergo changes. The author(s) and publisher have done everything possible to make this book accurate, up-to-date, and in accord with accepted standards at the time of publication. The author(s), editors, and publisher are not responsible for errors or omissions or for consequences from application of the book, and make no warranty, expressed or implied, in regard to the contents of the book. Any practice described in this book should be applied by the reader in accordance with professional standards of care used in regard to the unique circumstances that may apply in each situation. The reader is advised always to check product information (package inserts) for changes and new information regarding dose and contraindications before administering any drug. Caution is especially urged when using new or infrequently ordered drugs.

Library of Congress Cataloging-in-Publication Data

Riddle, Daniel L.
   Is this change real? : interpreting patient outcomes in physical therapy / Daniel L. Riddle, Paul W. Stratford.
      p. ; cm.
   Includes bibliographical references.
   ISBN 978-0-8036-2957-8
   I. Stratford, Paul W.   II. Title.
   [DNLM: 1. Physical Therapy Modalities.   2. Treatment Outcome. WB 460]

   615.8′2—dc23   2012047621

We'd like to dedicate this book to our wives. They may be short in stature (one reportedly stands 5′ 2¼″, which we believe to be an exaggeration) but their hearts are enormous. Don't know what we'd do without them.

Cheryl Cott, PhD
Professor
Department of Physical Therapy
University of Toronto
Toronto, Ontario, Canada

Eric Finstad, BHSc (PT), MSc (Sport Sci), FCAMPT
Physiotherapist
Killens Reid Physiotherapy
Ottawa, Ontario, Canada

John H. Hollman, PT, PhD
Director, Program in Physical Therapy, and Associate Professor
Department of Physical Medicine & Rehabilitation
Mayo Clinic
Rochester, Minnesota

Peter A. Huijbregts, PT, MSc, MHSc, DPT, OCS, FAAOMPT, FCAMT
Assistant Professor, Online Education
University of St. Augustine for Health Sciences
Victoria, British Columbia, Canada

Irene McEwen, PT, DPT, PhD, FAPTA
Professor
Department of Rehabilitation Sciences
University of Oklahoma Health Sciences Center
Oklahoma City, Oklahoma

Diane H. Pitts, PT, DPT, RN, BSN
Adjunct Instructor
Department of Physical Therapy
University of South Alabama
Mobile, Alabama

Ted J. Stevenson, MSc(PT)
Staff Physiotherapist
Rehabilitation Services
St. Boniface General Hospital
Winnipeg, Manitoba, Canada

Andrew J. Strubhar, PT, PhD
Associate Professor
Department of Physical Therapy and Health Science
Bradley University
Peoria, Illinois

Marianne Thornton, BScPT, MA (Human Kinetics), PhD candidate
Physiotherapist
Champlain Regional Stroke Program
Ottawa Hospital
Ottawa, Ontario, Canada

Frank B. Underwood, PT, PhD, ECS
Professor
Department of Physical Therapy
University of Evansville
Evansville, Indiana

Acknowledgments

Over the past three decades we have had the good fortune to work with and learn from many students, colleagues, and mentors. We are extremely grateful for their contributions to our lives. Without their support and encouragement, this book would not exist.

Contents

Chapter 5

What Does This Outcome Measurement Really Mean? *59*

Chapter 6

What Does a Change in the Outcome Measurement Indicate? *73*

Chapter 1

Outcome Assessment Is Not as Straightforward as It Appears

In a recent patient encounter, when asked how he was doing during follow-up, my patient told me the following: "I'm doing better but I still have some pain." At first blush, this may indicate some improvement, but does it really? These types of ambiguous responses are a real challenge for therapists making decisions about whether their patients are improving, getting worse, or staying the same. To achieve some clarity regarding his pain, when I asked him to rate his pain for the day, he scored it at a 5 on a 0 to 10 verbal pain rating scale. This score was 1 point less than the score reported on his initial evaluation about 2 weeks ago. What do I write in the medical record? How do I decide what to write? I want to capture the truth about the patient's condition, but I'm unclear on what the truth really is given his response to my question.

Dilemmas like this one are universal in physical therapy. When patients respond to questions like "How are you doing?" the risk of ambiguity rises. For example, the patient stated he was doing pretty well but he also noted his pain persisted. Does this mean he is getting better or does this mean his problems really have not changed in any meaningful way? Ambiguous responses are not isolated to patient self-reports of symptom status. Impairment measures and performance-based measures are also prone to ambiguity and error. For example, have you ever noticed when assessing a patient's grip strength or sitting posture that your findings vary with repeated testing? This book will help you to resolve

1

these types of unclear outcome assessments. We present clear outcome assessment and provide you with several clinically feasible approaches that will help you reduce the ambiguity inherent in all outcome measures.

Physical therapists are *the* recognized experts at quantifying health condition/disease consequences, setting meaningful patient-centered goals, choosing interventions to resolve patient problems, and assessing changes in outcome measures over time. This last step, using outcome measures to assess change, can appear to be deceptively simple on the surface. But as the example we posed at the beginning of the chapter illustrates, outcome assessment can be nuanced and difficult to interpret. The primary objectives of this book are to take full advantage of the outcomes literature and key conceptual frameworks to help you to (1) select outcome measures that are ideally suited to your patients' needs and (2) interpret outcome measures to optimize clinical decision making for individual patients. These objectives were driven by our understanding of and appreciation for outcome measurement. In short, our philosophical approach to outcome assessment is the following. The conscientious and judicious assessment of patients' outcomes is a complex clinical skill, much like patient assessment and treatment selection and delivery, and requires a conceptual framework and a specific body of knowledge.

We've written the book to be useful to clinicians and to educators. Outcome assessment is an essential, universal clinical skill that applies equally well to all areas of practice. No matter whether the patient is aged 1 day or 99 years or is affected by a neurological, cardiopulmonary, or musculoskeletal disorder, outcome assessment is essential to that patient's plan of care. It is our belief that clinicians practicing in all specialty areas will benefit by improving their understanding of outcome assessment and their sophistication in obtaining and interpreting outcome measurements. By applying the principles discussed in this text, we believe that clinicians will be able to better justify potential therapeutic effects of interventions for their patients and third-party payers.

We've also written the book for students and their instructors who will be able to apply the content across multiple courses in a curriculum. We believe that outcome assessment is an acquired high-level skill that requires time and effort to learn and apply. Much like examination and treatment, outcome assessment should, in our view, take on a central role in academic training. We would encourage educators to consider outcome assessment more broadly and not funnel the content into one course. We suggest, for example, that all instructors in neurological, musculoskeletal, and pediatrics courses consider adopting principles discussed in the book in their clinical courses. If students perceive these concepts to be essentials of routine practice that are independent of specialty area, it is our view that the principles are more likely to find their way into daily practice.

Some sections in the book that emphasize conceptual understanding and place less emphasis on more technical issues of measurement will be relatively light reading. You'll also find some sections in several chapters that are more technical in nature. This approach was driven by necessity. If you accept our premise that state-of-the-art outcomes assessment is an advanced clinical skill, then you will forgive us for including some technical (statistically driven) content in the book. For a clinician to take full advantage of the extensive literature on this topic, a small amount of technical content is necessary to understand the concepts and to take full advantage of this wealth of evidence-based information in clinical practice. We appreciate the aversion that many have toward this more technical (and admittedly drier) content. We have done our best to make this material reader friendly while at the same time acknowledging that some may be mildly intimidated by the equations, figures, and graphs. We encourage you to work through these sections of the book because we believe they will pay dividends for both you and your patients down the road.

We've set a very high bar, haven't we? We're going to provide you with the tools necessary to achieve these lofty objectives. But before outlining the content of the text, we will briefly introduce the requirements of an outcome measure, or more correctly, a standardized outcome measure.

▶ A Very Brief Introduction to Outcome Measures

Outcome measures must be proficient at discriminating among patients at a point in time and adept at assessing change over time. These two requirements are illustrated in the following sequence of events commonly observed in clinical practice. At a patient's initial assessment a physical therapist performs a number of tests and measures to determine the extent to which deficiencies exist. When a deficiency is identified, it is tracked over time to provide information about a patient's progress or deterioration. Typically, this is done by examining the change between the values of the previous and current assessments for the outcome of interest. A physical therapist's final decision is to determine whether or not a patient's target value has been met. At this stage, a challenge for the therapist is to select an optimal discrimination outcome measure: It must be adept at distinguishing between patients who have met their target goal and those who have not—more on this topic later in the book.

At this point you may be wondering what all the fuss over outcome measures has been over the past few decades. After all, doesn't simply asking patients how they are doing today and inquiring whether they have noticed a change since the previous visit meet the requirements? In a nutshell, the answer is yes, but there are a variety of reasons (elaborated on in the book) why this approach will potentially mislead therapists. As illustrated in the case scenario presented in the beginning of the chapter, broad questions like "How are you doing today?" are nonstandardized and can lead to ambiguous interpretation. Standardized outcome measures come equipped with formal descriptions of their conceptual framework and documentation of their development, application, and scoring. Moreover, standardized measures can be defended to the extent that their measurement properties within a defined context (e.g., condition, patient characteristics, setting, etc.) have been reported, critiqued, and substantiated in peer-reviewed forums. Standardized outcome measures are a necessary step in state-of-the-art outcome assessment.

▶ What's Ahead

We begin Chapter 2 of the book by providing summary descriptions of two conceptual frameworks that describe how outcome assessment fits into patient/client management. We emphasize the role of outcome assessment and summarize the various types of outcome measures in the context of the International Classification of Function, Disability and Health (ICF) model.[1] A major benefit of using the ICF model is that it frames outcomes assessment along a continuum (i.e., impairments, activity limitations, and participation restrictions), and we use this continuum to highlight the various types of outcomes assessments used by physical therapists. We also use the Hypothesis Oriented Algorithm for Clinicians (HOAC II) to describe outcome assessment in the context of a patient management model.[2,3] The HOAC II contributes to the discussion of outcomes assessment by providing an algorithm that incorporates a disablement model into patient management.

Chapter 3 builds on Chapter 2 by stimulating thought on how knowledge of the ICF and HOAC can be used to structure a comprehensive outcome assessment and form measurable goals from the information gained. This chapter also serves as a transition from the theoretical frameworks introduced in Chapter 2 to essential questions used to guide clinical decision making.

Chapters 4 through 8 provide therapists with a series of five questions that will assist in guiding decisions about which outcome measures to use and when to use them. We believe these five essential questions will provide therapists with an efficient way of navigating through the outcomes assessment literature to find outcome measures that are most likely to improve practice-based decisions. When we document the results of a measurement in the patient's medical record, we assume that the error associated with the measurement is small enough to not compromise the clinical decisions based on the value. Chapter 4 considers the question "How Confident Can I

Be About the Outcome Measurement on My Patient?" by linking fundamental concepts of reliability theory to confidence in clinical decisions. Specifically, this chapter provides a framework for conceptualizing measurement error in practical terms. Chapter 4 also illustrates how the results from reliability studies can be meaningfully applied in clinical practice.

With the exponential increase in available outcome measures over the past few decades it is not always obvious what a measured value means. To take the additional time associated with administering yet another measure in a busy practice setting, the measure's result must have meaning and provide more information with greater confidence than is available from the current assessment. In Chapter 5 we address the question "What Does This Outcome Measurement Really Mean?" by considering two component questions: (1) To what extent does the measure assess what it is intended to measure? (2) What is the interpretation of the measured value? The former question considers the extent to which one can draw valid inferences from a measurement, whereas the latter question addresses the extent to which qualitative meaning can be assigned to quantitative values.

In clinical practice it is often tempting to think of all change as being real change. In Chapters 1 through 5 we will have learned that error is associated with all measurements. Accordingly, it stands to reason that error is at play when considering the difference between the previous and current assessment values. Is a difference between measurements taken on two occasions likely to be real or merely an artifact of measurement error? If the change is real, is it clinically important? These are important questions when monitoring a patient's progress over the course of treatment. In Chapter 6 we introduce and compare three popularly applied methods to answer the question "What Does a Change in the Outcome Measurement Indicate?"

There's the old saying "If you don't know where you are going, you won't know when you get there." Patients frequently ask about their expected outcomes and physical therapists are expected not only to provide insightful answers to patients but also to document in the medical record the form of measurable long-term goals. In Chapter 7 we consider the question "How

Can I Establish a Target Goal Value for My Patient?" We describe five popular methods for establishing threshold values for goals.

In clinical practice, reassessments typically occur on a regular basis. The interval between assessments is often dictated by the complexity of the measurement process. For example, range of motion is often measured at each assessment for patients with limitations of movement. In contrast, more time-consuming tests such as the Berg Balance test or 6-minute walk test are likely to be reassessed at less frequent intervals. In Chapter 8 we consider the question "When Should Reassessments Take Place?" by introducing the concept that for each measure and patient there is an ideal reassessment interval that will minimize misclassification errors in the interpretation of a test result. By misclassification error we mean labeling a patient as having changed or not changed when the opposite is true.

We all know that use of standardized outcome measures requires staff and therapist commitment and that there are barriers to their routine use. Chapter 9 reviews frequently reported barriers to the successful implementation of standardized outcome measures in busy practice settings. We address barriers under the following headings: (1) barriers affecting the therapist, (2) barriers affecting the patient or patient/therapist interaction, and (3) resource and organizational barriers. This chapter goes on to suggest barrier-busting strategies for overcoming the identified barriers and for successfully implementing new outcome measures in your practice.

In Chapter 10, we provide a search strategy for locating outcome measures that may apply to a particular patient and we also present a succinct way of critiquing the quality of a group of similar measures in order to identify the optimal measure for a given patient or a given practice setting.

In Chapter 11, we provide two case reports. These reports illustrate how therapists might apply the concepts discussed in this book to individual patients.

The science of outcomes assessment has shown tremendous advances in the past few decades; like many scientific advances, such as those in diagnosis and intervention, cutting-edge outcomes assessment has not found its way into many clinical practice settings. As we indicated earlier in this chapter, it is our contention that outcomes assessment is an advanced clinical skill with its own evidence-based literature, much like diagnosis or treatment selection, and that patient care can be enhanced by the application of this new science to routine clinical practice. We hope that therapists will find the concepts in this book useful as they continue to work toward applying the latest scientific advances in outcomes assessment to their own clinical practices.

▪ Reference List

1. *International Classification of Functioning, Disability and Health: ICF.* Geneva, Switzerland: World Health Organization; 2001.
2. Rothstein JM, Echternach JL. Hypothesis-oriented algorithm for clinicians. A method for evaluation and treatment planning. *Phys Ther* 1986 September;66(9):1388–94.
3. Rothstein JM, Echternach JL, Riddle DL. The Hypothesis-Oriented Algorithm for Clinicians II (HOAC II): A guide for patient management. *Phys Ther* 2003 May;83(5):455–70.

Chapter 2

ICF and HOAC II: Two Conceptual Frameworks to Augment Clinical Practice

■ *Physicians spend the majority of their time diagnosing, treating, and preventing disease. Physical therapists, in contrast, spend most of their time diagnosing, treating, and preventing the consequences of disease. We are the go-to health-care experts for identifying and quantifying disease consequences and applying treatments to reduce or eliminate disease consequences to restore functional status. This chapter introduces (for those unfamiliar) or reviews (for those who are already familiar) two conceptual frameworks that go right to the heart of disease consequence diagnosis and outcome assessment.*

Two conceptual frameworks described in our literature are valuable tools for conceptualizing and then systematically addressing disease consequences in the course of physical therapy care. These frameworks are, in our opinion, useful to even the most seasoned clinicians. The frameworks have been around for many years and the current versions reflect state-of-the-art approaches to conceptualizing patient problems and how to solve them. Therapists spend many hours not only working with patients but also thinking about patients' disorders and how these disorders contributed to the patients' disablement. Restoring function (a key concept in the disablement process) is, after all, how we spend most of our professional time. The word disablement essentially describes the impact that disorders have on the functioning of body systems/organs, on basic person-level performance, and on functioning within society.[1] Even if you are familiar with these two frameworks, we urge you to review this chapter for an update. If these frameworks are new to you, we urge you to take some time to study this chapter more thoroughly because the remaining chapters in the book will build on many of the concepts introduced here.

What's Ahead

The purpose here is to review two conceptual frameworks that address a variety of issues related to outcome and the assessment of change in a patient's status. The first framework is the International Classification of Functioning, Disability and Health, or, if you prefer the much quicker version, the ICF.[2] The description of the disablement process in this framework has garnered worldwide acceptance, and for that reason, it is a framework that we should pay close attention to and, in our opinion, incorporate into our practices to the extent that we can. There is a lot to be said for a framework that describes the process by which patients seek medical care that has been accepted by all 191 member countries of the World Health Organization. There are very few issues that 191 countries could possibly agree on! Given this almost worldwide consensus, the ICF deserves our serious consideration.

The second framework that we will review in this chapter is the Hypothesis Oriented Algorithm for Clinicians (HOAC II).[3] This algorithm (or framework, if you like) has been in our literature under a previous name (HOAC) since 1986.[4] The original algorithm was introduced by Rothstein and Echternach in the following way:

> *To be useful, a conceptual scheme must guide the therapist in the use of evaluation for treatment planning and provide the therapist with a logical sequence of activities. To have widespread acceptance, this sequence must be independent of treatment philosophies; assist therapists in knowing when to seek aid from other health care professionals; and guide the processes of treatment planning, evaluation, and modification. (pg. 388)*

We believe that this same vision for why a framework is needed to help guide many practice-based decisions is as true today as it was more than two decades ago. Essentially, the newer version of HOAC was developed, in part, to incorporate a different but conceptually very similar disablement model to ICF, the Nagi model,[5] into the HOAC framework. This newer version of HOAC is creatively called HOAC II. Since one of us (DLR) helped to write this newer version, we reserve the right to poke fun at the lackluster and completely uncreative title!

We will first review the basic elements of the ICF disablement model and how these basic elements interact with one another. We will pay particular attention to defining the elements of the model and how these different elements relate to the assessment of treatment outcome and the assessment of patient change. We will describe and define the basic elements of HOAC II and elaborate on where and how therapists might assess outcome within the model. We also will rely on a few annotated case reports at the end of the book to help illustrate the applications of principles from both the ICF and HOAC II models because, after all, they are closely related, which is one of the reasons we are presenting both to begin the book! The final section of the chapter will discuss the melding of both the ICF and HOAC II into a comprehensive framework for patient problem solving. We view these two frameworks as complementary and, with the help of the rest of the book, we will discuss how they can be used together to assist you in determining whether apparent changes associated with your care are likely to be real and meaningful (to the patient and therapist), real (to the therapist) but meaningless (to the patient), or illusory (to everyone).

▶ The ICF Model of Disablement

The International Classification of Functioning, Disability and Health (ICF) is a comprehensive conceptual framework for describing the disablement process in a way that is generic and generalizable across countries and cultures. All 191 member countries of the World Health Organization have endorsed the ICF as the conceptual model for describing disablement in many contexts, including health and social policy and health care. As

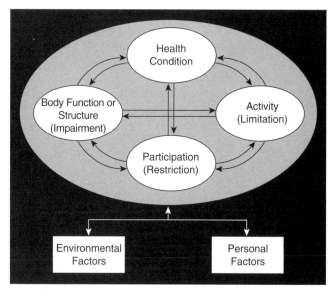

Figure 2-1 The International Classification of Functioning, Disability and Health (ICF) Conceptual Model

reported by Escorpizo and colleagues, the ICF also has been officially endorsed by the United Nations Statistical Office to track health and disability data around the world.[6] The ICF takes a comprehensive view of health from biological, personal, and social perspectives. The conceptual framework consists of several *dimensions* (see Fig. 2-1). The framework is biopsychosocial in nature with both function and disability being the final common pathway following interactions among the remaining dimensions in the model.

Key Elements of the ICF

There are six key dimensions that comprise the ICF conceptual framework (see Fig. 2-1). The dimension that usually initiates the disablement process in an individual patient is the *health condition.* This dimension describes the disease(s), disorder(s), injury(ies), aging, and congenital anomaly(ies) that potentially led the patient to seek care. These health conditions are very well known to us and include such disorders as stroke, pulmonary embolism, spinal stenosis, osteoarthritis, and so on.

The three dimensions that describe a continuum of human functioning are *body functions and structures, activity,* and *participation. Body functions and structures* describe human anatomical, physiological, and psychological functioning at the level of organs or organ systems. For example, a blood pressure measurement describes cardiovascular system function while a quadriceps femoris manual muscle test describes quadriceps muscle function. When, for example, cardiovascular or muscular structures or functions are abnormal (relative to what you would expect for the age- and gender-based population matched to your patient), then the patient is described as having an impairment in either cardiovascular function or quadriceps strength. Please see additional examples for each dimension within the ICF in Table 2-1.

Activity describes the execution of a task or action by the individual. These tasks or actions are generally described as being generic in nature without a clear connection to a societal context. For example, when we talk about person-level activities such as walking, sitting, standing, and reaching, we are talking about the person and not a specific organ or system, and we are not placing the action in a societal context. We are not, for example, talking about "sitting at work" or "standing at a religious service." Jette draws the useful distinction between *activity* and *participation* by describing *activity* as person-level actions that are examined generically in the clinic and not in the context of the patient's normal daily life.[7] When a person has a problem, for example with sitting or walking, the ICF describes this person as having an activity limitation. This definition of *activity* contrasts with the more complex participation dimension of the ICF.

Participation describes the person's involvement in life situations. In other words, the societal context is direct and obvious when discussing the *participation* dimension. Involvement with work or recreational situations entail participations and when, for example, people have difficulty with or are unable to perform their normal work or recreational activities, they are described

Table 2-1 Common Clinical Examples for Each Term in the ICF Disablement Model

ICF Dimension or Factor	A Few Common Clinical Examples
Health Condition	Stroke, fracture, spinal cord injury, torn meniscus, cerebral palsy, cancer
Body Function or Structure	Reduced quadriceps strength, reduced lung capacity, limited range of motion, spasticity, pain, altered sensation, feeling sad, being fearful, compromised balance
Activity	Abnormal gait pattern; altered ability to sit, stand, bend, reach, throw, carry, push, and basic personal care
Participation	Altered ability to work, prepare meals, clean house, socialize, exercise, attend group activities, attend school
Contextual Factor	
Environmental Factor	A person's physical workplace, attitudes of other persons, services available to the person
Personal Factor	A person's age, race, sex, fitness level, habits and lifestyle, social background and coping skills

as having a participation restriction in the ICF model. Table 2-2 provides a summary of the key terms from the ICF model and some straightforward examples for each term.

Finally, there are two additional key terms associated with the ICF classification system that we need to review and are crucial to understanding and applying the ICF model to daily practice. These two terms are described as contextual factors, presumably because they form the context of all that the person brings to daily life. The ICF describes two contextual factors: *personal factors* and *environmental factors*.

Environmental factors are the physical, social, and attitudinal environment in which people live. The ICF further defines environmental factors using several subdomains, such as support

Table 2-2 ICF Terms and Definitions

ICF Dimension or Factor	Definition	Term Used in the ICF to Describe a Problem or a Deficit
Health Condition	Disease, disorder, or injury	
Body Function or Structure	Physiological function of systems or anatomical parts of the body	Impairment
Activity	Execution of task or action by the person	Activity Limitation
Participation	Involvement in a life situation with a societal context	Participation Restriction
Contextual Factor	Complex background of a person's life	
Environmental Factor	Physical, social, and attitudinal environment of a person	Barrier or Facilitator
Personal Factor	Features of a person's particular background	Barrier or Facilitator

and relationships, attitudes and services, systems and policies. Table 2-3 provides several examples of each of these environmental factors. A quick glance at this table will reinforce the importance of considering environmental factors when planning a patient's care. Workplace environments and interactions, for example, often have a dramatic impact on a patient's plan of care and prognosis. As we've all seen in clinical practice, environmental factors can either serve as a barrier or as a facilitator to recovery, and the ICF recommends use of these terms to describe the potential impact of the various environmental factors on the disablement process.

The second contextual factor is termed *personal factors*; these are features of the person's particular background. Examples include gender, race/ethnicity, age, and comorbidities that are not part of the health condition for which the person is seeking

Table 2-3 Comprehensive List of Subdomains for ICF Terms from the ICF Conceptual Framework

ICF Dimension or Factor	Comprehensive List of ICF Subdomains
Health Condition	
Body Function	**1.** Mental functions
	2. Sensory functions and pain
	3. Voice and speech functions
	4. Functions of cardiovascular, haematological, immunologic, and respiratory systems.
	5. Functions of the digestive, metabolic, and endocrine systems
	6. Genitourinary and reproductive functions
	7. Neuromusculoskeletal and movement-related functions
	8. Functions of the skin and related structures
Body Structure	**1.** Structures of the nervous system
	2. The eye, ear, and related structures
	3. Structures involved in voice and speech
	4. Structures of the cardiovascular, immunologic and respiratory systems.
	5. Structures of the digestive, metabolic, and endocrine systems
	6. Structures of the genitourinary and reproductive systems
	7. Structures related to movement
	8. Skin and related structures
Activity	**1.** Learning and applying knowledge
	2. General tasks and demands
	3. Communication
	4. Mobility
	5. Self-care

Table 2-3	**Comprehensive List of Subdomains for ICF Terms from the ICF Conceptual Framework—cont'd**
ICF Dimension or Factor	**Comprehensive List of ICF Subdomains**
Participation	1. Domestic life
	2. Interpersonal interactions and relationships
	3. Major life areas
	4. Community, social, and civic life
Contextual Factor	
Environmental Factor	1. Products and technology in the environment
	2. Natural environment and human-made changes to the environment
	3. Support and relationships of people in the environment
	4. Attitudes of people in the environment
	5. Services, systems, and policies of the environment
Personal Factor	(Not specifically characterized in the ICF) Examples include age, sex, race/ethnicity, health conditions, fitness level, habits, lifestyle, social background, life experiences, coping skills and styles

care. It is blatantly obvious to say that these factors have an impact on outcome. In our opinion, the critical personal and environmental factors that therapists need to pay closest attention to are those that are modifiable. We can do nothing about a patient's age, for example, but we can definitely modify a patient's workplace in order to positively impact the disablement process (more on this topic when we get to HOAC II). Table 2-3 provides a complete summary of the subcategories under the dimensions and factors that comprise the ICF model. As you can see from this table, the ICF addresses all major sources and serves as a comprehensive way to characterize the disablement process in all patients no matter the health condition.

As Figure 2-1 illustrates, the relationships among the various dimensions and contextual factors are complex. The older version of the ICF (the International Classification of Impairments, Disabilities and Handicaps—ICIDH) suggested a linear and sequential relationship: A disorder led to an impairment which led to an activity limitation and then participation restriction. As we know, the disablement process is not a clean sequential process, but rather a complex one with multiple interactions among dimensions and contextual factors (as indicated by the arrows pointed in multiple directions in the figure). In clinical practice this rather clean conceptual framework illustrated in Figure 2-1 plays out in a more complex and somewhat random way (on the surface). Our role as rehabilitation experts is to attempt to sort out these arrows in the process of finding solutions to patients' problems. We will discuss more on this later when we talk about interfacing the HOAC II and the ICF frameworks.

ICF-Based Methods for Assessing Outcome

The ICF serves as a clearly defined model for characterizing outcome measures that may be used to assess the change in patients receiving physical therapy interventions. The outcomes that are likely the most proximate to the types of interventions used by physical therapists are body function and structure outcomes. Given physical therapists' emphasis on measuring disease consequences, we spend much of our time during the examination quantifying the extent of our patients' impairments. And we are extremely good at measuring impairments. We spend a lot of time on this because many of our interventions are directed specifically toward resolving impairments.

For example, for patients with adhesive capsulitis of the shoulder, we spend a great deal of time in treatment attempting to restore glenohumeral range of motion, accessory motion, and movement-related impairments of the scapulothoracic joint. We also spend time resolving inflammation and pain in these patients. For patients with cardiovascular or pulmonary disorders, our treatments are many times focused on restoring pulmonary or cardiac function. Much of our time is spent resolving impairments, no matter the age or the disorder of our patients. Given this heavy emphasis on impairment resolution, it is no surprise we take multiple measures of impairments during the plan of care. Some impairments are highly important and have direct relevance to patients, such as pain. Most impairments, however, while potentially important, may not be relevant to the patient. The major limitations of impairment measurements are that they may only be weakly related or potentially not related at all to why patients sought care for their problems.

We therefore encourage a greater emphasis on outcomes that more closely resemble daily function and, ideally, directly relate to why the patient sought care in the first place. The ICF dimensions that would have the greatest utility (because they directly measure person-level function and not organ or system-level function) are the outcome measures that capture either the activity or participation dimensions. We now have many outcome measures from the activity or participation dimensions at our disposal and more are being developed because the research and clinical community has recognized the importance of capturing outcome at the person level.

Table 2-4 summarizes some of the more common outcome measures used by physical therapists. A quick look at the table will indicate that many of our activity limitation measures are measurements of the actual performance of such various activities as walking, stair climbing, or getting up out of a chair. Participation restrictions, on the other hand, are usually measured using a paper-and-pencil or computer-based interface because it is not practical for us to observe patients actually interacting in societal contexts. While we can observe and even use our stopwatches or other measurement approaches on patients while walking or stair climbing, for example, it is not practical for most of us to use a similar approach for patients while they are working or attending a social activity. Even given this limitation, most agree that patient-centered care mandates the use of measures that capture the highest level of human

Table 2-4	Common Clinical Examples of Outcome Measurements for Each Term in the ICF Disablement Model
Dimension or Factor	**A Few Common Outcome Measures**
Health Condition	Blood culture for infection, MRI or radiographic findings for fracture or soft tissue disease, ultrasonic imaging of heart function, surgical finding, cluster of signs and symptoms indicative of disease process without other diagnostic gold standard (e.g., fibromyalgia)
Body Function or Structure	Manual muscle test grade or dynamometer score, goniometric measurement, forced expiratory volume, VAS pain measurement, deep tendon reflex score, sensation test, fear avoidance behavior questionnaire score, Berg balance test score
Activity	20-meter or 400-meter walk test, sitting test score, AM-PAC Mobility Scale,[9–11] get up and go test, stair climbing test, Short Physical Performance Battery,[12] Bayley Scales of Infant Development[13]
Participation	Single-item questions related to work or recreational performance, Ab-IAP,[14] Lymph-ICF,[15] The Participation Scale[16]
Contextual Factor Environmental Factor	Measurement of a person's physical workplace, attitudes of other persons, services available to the person
Personal Factor	Measurement of a person's fitness level, habits and lifestyle, social background and coping skills

functioning, the activity limitations and participation restrictions that are most problematic for our patients.[8] Most commonly, we rely on self-report measures in lieu of actual performance measures to capture the participation restriction domain in our patients.

The developmental history of self-reported paper-and-pencil–based outcome measures began long before the current ICF model was proposed. Some of our more commonly used measures therefore lacked a clear conceptual framework when they were being developed. The Roland and Morris Questionnaire (RMQ) for low back pain, for example, was developed in 1983. As you might expect, this scale and many others were not grounded in a clearly articulated conceptual framework and therefore combined two or more dimensions into one scale. While scales like the RMQ are still commonly used and clearly have utility in daily practice, they can potentially provide difficult-to-interpret scores, given that they contain items that mix impairments, activity limitations, and participation restrictions. For example, the RM scale contains this item: "My back or leg is painful almost all of the time," which captures an impairment, albeit an important one. Another item—"I walk more slowly than usual because of my back and/or leg pain"—captures an activity limitation. A third item—"I avoid heavy jobs around the house because of my back and/or leg pain"—is more closely aligned with a participation restriction because it involves a social context.

We refer to scales like the RM scale as "hybrid" scales because they are not designed with a specific disablement-based conceptual framework. It may be difficult to describe what the RM score means because different items represent different conceptual meanings when considering the ICF. While these scales are still in common use and still provide potentially useful information, we suspect that, over time, more conceptually clear scales will gain acceptance and replace these "hybrid" measures.

Disablement Examples Using the ICF

The ICF can be used to clearly characterize the disablement process in an albeit simplistic but, it is hoped, helpful way. The examples in Tables 2-5 to 2-7 provide a quick and easy way to "put the ICF pieces together" to provide the reader with big-picture view of the disablement processes for a variety of patients. Each of the following examples briefly illustrates just a few of the key consequences of the health condition.

Table 2-5 Example: Applying ICF to a Person with Spinal Cord Injury

Example #1: This patient was involved in a motor vehicle accident resulting in a spinal cord injury. The patient is currently being seen in an acute care setting

Health Condition	Body Structure or Function Impairment	Activity Limitation	Participation Restriction
Thoracic spinal cord injury	Lower extremity muscle paralysis, lower extremity anesthesia	Unable to sit independently, unable to ambulate, unable to self-care	Unable to work, unable to do recreational activities, unable to participate in social activities

Key environmental factors: support system, attitudes of family and friends, housing situation

Key personal factors: age, socioeconomic status, coping style, fitness, previous health conditions

We indicated earlier that these examples are most likely dramatic oversimplifications of an oftentimes complex disablement process. However, we believe that they serve as clear, simple examples to reinforce the concepts of ICF in a way that at least begins to approximate clinical practice. In all examples, one can imagine the need for outcome measures for each dimension of the disablement process. In our view, the greatest need for outcome measures concerns the activity limitation and participation restriction dimensions of the ICF. These dimensions capture person-level functions and it is these dimensions that align directly with most of the reasons that patients seek health care. For this reason, we spend most of the remainder of the book talking about outcome measures for activity limitations and participation restrictions.

With that said, we also acknowledge the importance of body structure and function impairments. These measures are

Table 2-6 Example: Applying ICF to a Person with Low Back Pain

Example #2: This patient was diagnosed with a herniated disk in the lumbar spine and is seeking physical therapy for his low back and left leg pain.

Health Condition	Body Structure or Function Impairment	Activity Limitation	Participation Restriction
Herniated disk in the lumbar spine	Left-sided low back, posterior buttock, thigh and calf pain, reduced lumbar flexion, positive straight leg raise on left	Unable to sit without pain, unable to pick up objects off the floor, unable to stand for prolonged periods	Unable to complete tasks at work, unable to exercise, unable to sit during religious services

Key environmental factors: work environment, attitudes of family

Key personal factors: age, socioeconomic status, coping style, fitness, lifestyle, previous health conditions

ubiquitous in physical therapy practice and are of critical importance when formulating hypotheses about the causes of patients' problems. "Causes" in this context relate to disease consequences and extend beyond the usually simple and relatively uninformative (in the context of physical therapy treatment formulation) health condition diagnostic labels.

Outcome assessment may also apply to the health condition, but in this case, the "outcome" of interest is the presence or absence of the disorder that is hypothesized to be present. When we are unsure about the presence of a health condition we may request or refer the patient for additional diagnostic testing to either support or refute the presence of a hypothesized health condition. In this case, the outcome measurement would be the diagnostic test results. For example, the radiographic findings

Table 2-7 Example Applying ICF to a Person with Pulmonary Disease

Example #3: This patient was diagnosed with chronic obstructive pulmonary disease and is seeking physical therapy to improve her functional status.

Health Condition	Body Structure or Function Impairment	Activity Limitation	Participation Restriction
COPD	Reduced pulmonary function, shortness of breath on exertion, reduced lower extremity strength, fear of activity, compromised balance	Unable to walk more than 50 feet without fatigue, unable to climb a flight of steps	Unable to visit friends outside of the home, unable to walk in the park

Key environmental factors: support system, attitudes of family and friends, housing situation, medical technology availability, community services

Key personal factors: age, socioeconomic status, coping style, fitness and lifestyle, previous health conditions

for a patient suspected of having a fracture could serve as a validated outcome measure for either the presence or absence of fracture. Outcome assessment for health conditions is not discussed further in this book because we are primarily interested in outcome measures that require reassessment, such as body structure or function impairments, activity limitations, or participation restrictions—outcomes therapists routinely reassess on their patients.

We hope you now have a general understanding of the ICF model and can see some potential advantages to applying the ICF as an overarching conceptual model to guide clinical practice. We will now discuss the second conceptual framework that we mentioned at the beginning of the chapter, the Hypothesis Oriented Algorithm for Clinicians II.

▶ The HOAC II

The HOAC II[17] is a fairly substantial modification of the original HOAC,[18–19] which was designed to be a patient-centered conceptual framework for guiding patient management. HOAC II was written and published in response to the increased popularity of disablement models[5,20] and to the many changes in the health-care environment that ensued over the approximately 20 years since the publication of the original HOAC.

HOAC II is a conceptual model that suggests a process a therapist could apply while managing a patient's problems. The model consists of two parts: (1) Part 1 leads the therapist through clinical decision making from the medical history to the intervention; (2) Part 2 is a reassessment algorithm designed to assist the therapist in identifying potential deficiencies in the treatment plan when patient response to treatment is less than optimal. The HOAC II model can be used to guide documentation or it may simply serve as a guide to some of the reasoning that goes on and actions that are taken during a plan of care. We by no means believe that HOAC II needs to be followed verbatim. We've seen too many of our ideas go belly up to believe that HOAC II is the best or only approach to follow when treating patients. Rather, we hope that clinicians reading this book and reviewing HOAC II will find some value in the framework and, in the process of treating patients, that some aspect of HOAC II added a level of clarity to the always challenging process of treating patients.

We understand and appreciate that some therapists may have no interest in HOAC II. The good news is that concepts reviewed in the following few pages apply no matter the conceptual framework a therapist uses to guide examination and treatment. In other words, we ask that you keep reading because we believe that you may still find some valuable nuggets even if you are not interested in the general approach.

Key Elements of HOAC II

The conceptual framework for HOAC II is nicely summarized in the following four figures (Figs. 2-2 to 2-4); we will describe

Text continued on page 29

Hypothesis-Oriented Algorithm for Clinicians II
(HOAC II – PART 1)

Collect Initial Data
From: referral information, the medical record, observation before any formal evaluation is begun, and the interview

↓

Generate Patient-Identified Problems (PIPs) List
Problems listed are almost exclusively descriptions of functional limitations and disabilities. Problems are described solely in patient-oriented terms reflecting the patient's views of what he or she can and cannot do.

↓

Formulate Examination Strategy
Strategy is based on an initial set of hypotheses generated from available data and the nature of the patient-identified problems.

Consultation if needed

Conduct the Examination, Analyze Data, Refine Hypotheses, and Carry Out Additional Examination Procedures Needed to Confirm or Deny Hypotheses

↓

Add Non–Patient-Identified Problems (NPIPs) to the Problem List
These problems are not identified by the patient. NPIPs are identified by the therapist and others working with the patient (this could include family members). NPIPs are often anticipated problems, which if not prevented from occuring, will lead to disability and diminished health status.

For Each Existing Problem | For Each Anticipated Problem

Generate a Hypothesis (or Hypotheses) as to Why the Problem Exists
Hypotheses often represent the identification of a level of impairment thought to be causing a problem. Sometimes hypotheses may be the identification of pathological processes causing impairments, functional limitations, or disabilities. All hypotheses must be verifiable through obtainable measurements.

Identify the Rationale
(by use of theoretical arguments or by use of data)
For Believing Anticipated Problems Are Likely to Occur Unless Intervention Is Provided

The justification (rationale) for treating anticipated problems is the case (argument) as to why pathologies or impairments will lead to functional limitations and disabilities unless intervention is provided.

Consultation if needed | Consultation if needed

→ **Go To "Refine Problem List"** ←

Figure 2-2 **HOAC II–Part 1:** Hypothesis-Oriented Algorithm for Clinicians II. With permission of the American Physical Therapy Association. This material is copyrighted, and any further reproduction or distribution requires written permission from APTA.

HOAC II – PART 2 (Anticipated Problems)

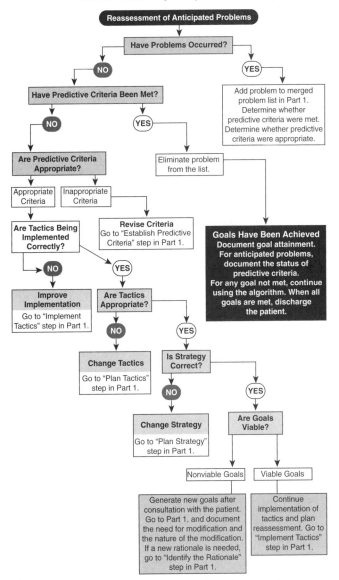

Figure 2-3 **HOAC II–Part 2:** Anticipated Problems. With permission of the American Physical Therapy Association. This material is copyrighted, and any further reproduction or distribution requires written permission from APTA.

HOAC II – PART 2 (Existing Problems)

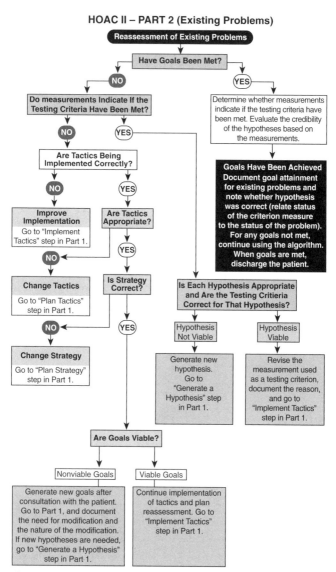

Figure 2-4 **HOAC II–Part 2:** Existing Problems. With permission of the American Physical Therapy Association. This material is copyrighted, and any further reproduction or distribution requires written permission from APTA.

some of the key elements here. For a more comprehensive description, we encourage you to read the original description[21] and the accompanying case report that describes the use of HOAC II with a patient with low back pain.[22]

HOAC II acknowledges that there are two types of problems reported by patients (see Fig. 2-2). First are those problems present at the time of care and that require intervention. Patients may, for example, voice a concern about an inability to ambulate without a limp. The second type of problems are those that may occur in the future if no intervention is provided to reduce the risk of occurrence. For example, a patient who has had a stroke may be concerned about a future risk of pain and reduced function of the shoulder involved. Prevention and the provision of preventive interventions is a cornerstone of sound physical therapy care; HOAC II has incorporated methods to justify and to subsequently test for the soundness of delivering preventive interventions.

Because current problems and potential future problems are fundamentally different in terms of management and outcome assessment, both are dealt with differently in HOAC II. These two types of problems are termed **existing problems** and **anticipated problems**. Patient problems may be reported by the patient (**patient-identified problems—PIPs**) or they may be perceived by others, including the therapist, and these are termed **non-patient-identified problems—NPIPs**. Existing problems may be PIPs or NPIPs, and anticipated problems may also be PIPs or NPIPs.

Hypotheses, in the context of HOAC II, are a therapist's assessments of the most likely causes of the patient's problems. Patient problems relate, in most cases, to the activity limitations and participation restrictions that led the patient to seek or require care. In the HOAC II causes of problems do not relate to the more traditional biomedical approach to identifying disease or causes of disease. Rather, causes in the context of physical therapy care relate most commonly to causes of disease consequences. For most patients, the key disease consequences are the impairments that preclude the patient from accomplishing what she or he would like to do. In addition, modifiable contextual factors may also contribute to patient problems and require attention from the therapist. In short, the focus is not on the disease per se but rather on disease consequences, the key impairments that have resulted, and any modifiable contextual factors that serve as barriers to recovery. Rarely, a patient may be seen in whom the therapist suspects a previously undiagnosed disorder. In this case, the hypothesis may identify a previously undiagnosed disease, and this would warrant referral to a physician for work-up to determine if the suspected disorder is present.

For **existing problems**, HOAC II attempts to apply the scientific method to the process of patient care by using **testing criteria** to determine whether the hypotheses about causes of patient problems are likely correct. Therapists define the **testing criteria** that will be used to judge whether the key impairments that are leading to functional loss actually were important (e.g., reduced muscle force of the scapular adductors leading to reduced shoulder function in a patient with impingement syndrome). If the intervention improves scapular adductor strength, the patient's function should improve. If not, the hypothesis is likely incomplete or incorrect and the therapist can take corrective action.

In terms of **anticipated problems**, we are talking about those that may occur in the future if corrective action is not taken. Because we are talking about potential future events, we cannot in most cases actually document that we prevented a negative outcome. Hypotheses for existing problems, in contrast, can be formally tested because a change in the variables of interest can be measured. This is not the case for anticipated problems. There is no observable change, because the events we are trying to prevent will only occur in the future, if they occur at all. In addition, even without a preventive intervention, a problem may not arise in the future. The HOAC II, therefore, defines **predictive criteria** for **anticipated problems** (see Fig. 2-3).

Predictive criteria are target levels of measurements, behaviors, or knowledge that need to be demonstrated by the patient in order to provide evidence that a preventive intervention has a reasonable chance of preventing a future event. For example, when trying to prevent skin breakdown on a patient with a spinal cord injury, the following could serve as predictive criteria for a preventive intervention aimed at reducing risk of future skin breakdown: (1) performance of wheelchair pushups a given number of times per hour and (2) the patient or someone else monitoring the skin at specified intervals. The key is that **predictive criteria** need to be observable and ideally not just an expression by the patient of an increased awareness. Available evidence should always be used as a basis for selection of testing and predictive criteria.

Part 2 of HOAC II concerns methods for reassessment. There are two algorithms, one for **existing problems** and one for **anticipated problems**. These reassessment algorithms are designed for those times when patients do not appear to be responding to a treatment plan. Part 2 takes the therapist through a series of questions designed to alert them to various aspects of the intervention that may not be optimal. A potential benefit of HOAC II is that it requires all treatments to be linked directly to **hypotheses** so that no treatment will be provided unless it addresses the key impairments or modifiable contextual factors identified in the **hypotheses**. We will leave it to you to explore further by reading the published paper on HOAC II or by studying the accompanying figures of the HOAC II conceptual framework.

Outcomes Assessment Using HOAC II

Outcomes assessment, in the context of HOAC II falls under three major categories: (1) outcomes related to testing criteria and predictive criteria, (2) outcomes related to goal achievement, and (3) outcomes related to the medical diagnosis. Changes in the impairments comprising the testing criteria require reassessment to determine if the key impairments are showing progression toward the thresholds established in the testing criteria. Ideally, the impairments show a trend toward improvement as the patient moves toward accomplishing the goals. Of course, this may not be the case, which is why assessment of both the key impairments and the goals is important.

The same is true for the predictive criteria established for anticipated problems.

With HOAC II, the therapist develops a strategy for outcomes assessment by deciding on a time interval for reassessing the patient's status. Therapists should have a reasonable idea as to when key impairments, activity limitations, and participation restrictions may show change (see more on this concept in Chapter 6). These temporally driven changes are likely to be different for different patients and are influenced, to a great extent, by the patient's prognosis. Testing criteria outcomes are assessed after a period of time during which the therapist would have reasonably expected the patient's condition to change, at least to some extent.

Similarly, assessment for activity limitations and participation restrictions should occur when change is reasonably likely and not necessarily at each visit. Some clinics may require patients to complete self-report measures at every visit. Given that the likelihood for change after one visit may be very low for some patients, reassessment over such a short interval may not be optimal and in some cases could lead to erroneous impressions of change.

Outcomes related to the medical diagnosis are likely only to be relevant when the therapist refers the patient for medical work-up to assess for a previously undiagnosed disorder. The reassessment interval in this case is driven by the time taken to complete the work-up. The outcome will be either a confirmation of the therapist's suspicion or a confirmation that the patient does not have the disorder.

▶ Blending ICF and HOAC II

HOAC II was developed, in part, to align with the more contemporary disablement models.[5,20,23] It is therefore a simple task to link the ICF and HOAC II models and to provide a few examples of how this might be done. The advantages of such a linkage are many. One of the many barriers to improving practice is the use of many different sets of terminology and jargon when describing practice and the underlying bases for clinical decisions. By using the HOAC II and ICF frameworks in combination, clinicians would be able to communicate clearly regarding rationale and approach. We understand that this is "pie in the sky," but even a slight realignment to these frameworks would, at a minimum, improve our chances to enhance communication among therapists and clinics and, potentially, worldwide, given the broad acceptance of the ICF. It also is our opinion that these frameworks can potentially improve practice in other ways. The HOAC II is grounded in the scientific method and ICF clearly defines disablement in a way that is universally accepted. This would appear to be an ideal combination and, at least in theory, should improve the standard of care. We both agree, however, that research is needed to provide evidence of enhanced utility for either of these frameworks.

One of us published a case report using HOAC II;[24] the skeletal framework of this case report is summarized in Figure 2-5. We have attempted to provide summary information for each step in the HOAC II Part 1 algorithm and, along with the patient information, we have provided a link to corresponding ICF disablement terms. Figure 2-5 summarizes the outcomes using individual items reported by the patient. Figure 2-6 offers an alternative to the use of patient-reported individual activity limitations and participation restrictions. This figure provides scores for self-report measures that could serve as alternative measures of activity limitations and participation restrictions.

Either method has potential value. In our view, the strength of the first method is that it identifies specific patient-reported items that presumably were most important to the patient. The limitation of this approach is that when a small number of items are identified, there is a risk of missing true change, given that error increases as the number of items sampled is reduced. The other limitation of this approach is that the therapist will typically ask patients directly about their problematic activities. Patients may be prone to providing biased responses, depending on their perceived need to please (or not) the therapist providing the care. The strengths of the second method are many and are the major impetus for the remaining chapters of this book. The

Text continued on page 36

The HOAC II - Part 1

	Patient Data	Corresponding ICF Disablement Terms
Collect Initial Data		
PIPS List	Unable to roll in bed, bend forward, slouch, sit without pain, sleep uninterrupted, don stockings	Activity limitations
	Unable to do yard work, exercise, or ride bicycle without pain, compromised productivity at work	Participation restrictions
Examination Strategy		
Conduct Examination	Limited and painful trunk flexion, extension, lumbar accessory motion, limited hamstring length	Impairments
NPIPS List	Work-related psychological distress and prolonged sitting at work, limited hamstring muscle length	Contextual factors
Generate Hypotheses	PIPS due to L3–L5 area inflammation and flexion, extension and accessory motion impairments; NPIPS contributing to problems	Activity limitations and participation restrictions linked to impairments and contextual factors
Identify Rationale for Anticipated Problems		
Merge and Refine Problem Lists	To move in bed, forward bend, slouch, sit, and sleep without pain, don stockings without pain	Goals—activity limitations
Establish Goals	Do yard work, exercise, and ride bicycle, normal productivity at work	Goals—partic. restrictions
	Minimize risk of future low back pain	Contextual factors
Establish Testing Criteria	110 degrees of forward bending, 25 degrees of backward bending, accessory motion WNL and all without pain	Target levels—impairments from hypothesis
Establish Predictive Criteria	Patient report of reduced work-related stress and use of new routine for prevention of prolonged sitting, SLR to 80 degrees bilaterally	Target levels—contextual factors from NPIPS
Plan Intervention Strategy and Tactics		

Figure 2-5 Summary of HOAC II Elements, Patient Data and Corresponding ICF Terms from Previous Published Case Report.[19] Adapted with permission of the American Physical Therapy Association. This material is copyrighted, and any further reproduction or distribution requires written permission from APTA.

34

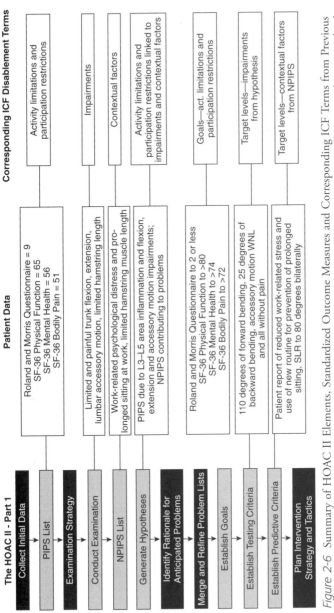

Figure 2-6 Summary of HOAC II Elements, Standardized Outcome Measures and Corresponding ICF Terms from Previous Published Case Report.[19] Adapted with permission of the American Physical Therapy Association. This material is copyrighted, and any further reproduction or distribution requires written permission from APTA.

Roland and Morris scale, for example, has been used extensively in the literature and we know how to interpret baseline, discharge, and change scores. We know how much change is necessary to make inferences about whether the change may be real,[25] and whether the final score may be indicative of someone who has recovered from low back pain.[26] The remaining chapters will discuss various issues related to the use of standardized outcome measures and the potential advantages of standardized outcome measures in daily practice.

▪ Reference List

1. Verbrugge LM, Jette AM. The disablement process. *Soc Sci Med* 1994 January;38(1):1–14.

2. World Health Organization. *International Classification of Functioning, Disability and Health: ICF.* Geneva: World Health Organization; 2001.

3. Rothstein JM, Echternach JL, Riddle DL. The Hypothesis-Oriented Algorithm for Clinicians II (HOAC II): A guide for patient management. *Phys Ther* 2003;83(5):455–70.

4. Rothstein JM, Echternach JL. Hypothesis-oriented algorithm for clinicians. A method for evaluation and treatment planning. *Phys Ther* 1986;66(9):1388–94.

5. Nagi SZ. An epidemiology of disability among adults in the United States. *Milbank Mem Fund Q Health Soc* 1976;54(4):439–67.

6. Escorpizo R, Stucki G, Cieza A, Davis K, Stumbo T, Riddle DL. Creating an interface between the International Classification of Functioning, Disability and Health and physical therapist practice. *Phys Ther* 2010; 90(7):1053–63.

7. Jette AM. Toward a common language for function, disability, and health. *Phys Ther* 2006;86(5):726–34.

8. Bergeson SC, Dean JD. A systems approach to patient-centered care. *JAMA* 2006 20;296(23):2848–51.

9. Haley SM, Coster WJ, Andres PL, et al. Activity outcome measurement for postacute care. *Med Care* 2004;42(1 Suppl):I49–I61.

10. Haley SM, Siebens H, Coster WJ, et al. Computerized adaptive testing for follow-up after discharge from inpatient rehabilitation: I. Activity outcomes. *Arch Phys Med Rehabil* 2006;87(8):1033–42.

11. Siebens H, Andres PL, Pengsheng N, Coster WJ, Haley SM. Measuring physical function in patients with complex medical and postsurgical conditions: A computer adaptive approach. *Am J Phys Med Rehabil* 2005;84(10):741–8.

12. Guralnik JM, Ferrucci L, Pieper CF, et al. Lower extremity function and subsequent disability: Consistency across studies, predictive models, and value of gait speed alone compared with the short physical performance battery. *J Gerontol A Biol Sci Med Sci* 2000;55(4): M221–M231.

13. Gollenberg AL, Lynch CD, Jackson LW, McGuinness BM, Msall ME. Concurrent validity of the parent-completed Ages and Stages Questionnaires, 2nd Ed. with the Bayley Scales of Infant Development II in a low-risk sample. *Child Care Health Dev* 2010;36(4):485–90.

14. Pollard B, Dixon D, Dieppe P, Johnston M. Measuring the ICF components of impairment, activity limitation and participation restriction: An item analysis using classical test theory and item response theory. *Health Qual Life Outcomes* 2009;7:41.

15. Devoogdt N, Van KM, Geraerts I, Coremans T, Christiaens MR. Lymphoedema Functioning, Disability and Health Questionnaire (Lymph-ICF): Reliability and validity. *Phys Ther* 2011;91(6): 944–57.

16. van Brakel WH, Anderson AM, Mutatkar RK, et al. The Participation Scale: Measuring a key concept in public health. *Disabil Rehabil* 2006;28(4):193–203.

17. Rothstein JM, Echternach JL, Riddle DL. The Hypothesis-Oriented Algorithm for Clinicians II (HOAC II): A guide for patient management. *Phys Ther* 2003;83(5):455–70.

18. Echternach JL, Rothstein JM. Hypothesis-oriented algorithms. *Phys Ther* 1989;69(7):559–64.

19. Rothstein JM, Echternach JL. Hypothesis-oriented algorithm for clinicians. A method for evaluation and treatment planning. *Phys Ther* 1986;66(9):1388–94.

20. World Health Organization. *International Classification of Functioning, Disability and Health: ICF.* Geneva, Switzerland: World Health Organization; 2001.

21. Rothstein JM, Echternach JL, Riddle DL. The Hypothesis-Oriented Algorithm for Clinicians II (HOAC II): A guide for patient management. *Phys Ther* 2003;83(5):455–70.

22. Riddle DL, Rothstein JM, Echternach JL. Application of the HOAC II: An episode of care for a patient with low back pain. *Phys Ther* 2003; 83(5):471–85.

23. Verbrugge LM, Jette AM. The disablement process. *Soc Sci Med* 1994; 38(1):1–14.

24. Riddle DL, Rothstein JM, Echternach JL. Application of the HOAC II: An episode of care for a patient with low back pain. *Phys Ther* 2003; 83(5):471–85.

25. Stratford PW, Binkley J, Solomon P, Finch E, Gill C, Moreland J. Defining the minimum level of detectable change for the Roland-Morris questionnaire. *Phys Ther* 1996;76(4):359–65.

26. Kamper SJ, Maher CG, Herbert RD, Hancock MJ, Hush JM, Smeets RJ. How little pain and disability do patients with low back pain have to experience to feel that they have recovered? *Eur Spine J* 2010;19(9): 1495–501.

Merging the ICF and HOAC with Outcome Assessment

Physical therapists focus much of their attention toward restoring a patient's functional status. However, a substantial amount of time also is spent screening for previously undiagnosed disease and measuring the extent of impairment. Therefore, there are many times when therapists include impairment and disease-related measures as well as person-level measures of activity limitation and participation restriction during outcome assessment.

Thus far, this book has examined outcome assessment from a broad perspective and, in the context of the theoretical frameworks presented in Chapter 2, outcome measures cover the gamut from disease status, to physical and psychosocial impairment, to person-level activity limitation and participation restriction. Of critical importance is the concept that these various outcome measures are not necessarily strongly related to one another. When we measure one outcome, for example, joint range of motion physical impairment, this measurement should not serve as a surrogate for a different ICF domain, for example, activity limitation.

A strong argument can be made for measuring multiple ICF domains during a plan of care. Hypotheses guiding treatment planning, for example, may focus on restoring strength and range of motion, say, in a patient with low back pain or spinal cord injury. Strength and range-of-motion impairment measures provide critical information to guide the therapist in determining the potential impact of their interventions on these presumably important impairments resulting from the inciting disease or injury. However, the relationship between these impairment measures and the patient's activity limitations or participation restrictions is likely not very strong. For example, Hazard and colleagues found that the Pearson product moment correlation between strength and ROM impairments and dis- ability as measured with the Oswestry Low Back Pain and Disability Questionnaire[1] was 0.40 for men and 0.52 for women.[2] Correlations among pain and ROM impairment mea- sures were also in this moderate range. These data suggest that physical impairment, pain, and disability outcome measures for patients with low back pain capture different attributes of a patient's recovery and cannot be used as substitutes for each other.

Similar moderate associations between physical impairment measures and person-level activity limitation or participation restriction have been found for a variety of disorders. For example, Rantanen and colleagues found that knee extensor strength explained only 42.3% of the variation in maximum walking speed in elderly women with a variety of disorders.[3] In addition, relationships among physical impairments such as strength and ROM and activity limitations such as gait speed are not as straightforward as they may appear. Sometimes they demonstrate a nonlinear relationship, suggesting that one should not assume a more straightforward linear relationship among impairment and disability.[4] The take-home message from this substantial body of literature examining relationships among ICF domains is that these domains are typically only moderately related and sometimes related in a complex, nonlinear way. Our view based on this literature is that outcome measures of one domain should not be assumed to adequately represent outcome measures of another domain and that therapists should routinely obtain outcome measures from multiple ICF domains during a plan of care.

In this book we are encouraging the use of the HOAC II in combination with ICF to shape your outcome assessment, and as the previous discussion suggests, we are encouraging a comprehensive outcome assessment that addresses multiple domains of the ICF. Ultimately, what typically is most important in patient care, and what is typically addressed when setting goals for care, is the patient's functional status. When it comes to goal setting, we encourage the use of **SMART** goals, which we define as goals that provide a **S**pecific description of the outcome of interest; are **M**easurable; are **A**ttainable given the unique characteristics of a patient, the desired amount of change, and the anticipated effectiveness of the intervention; are **R**elevant to the patient primarily but also the physical therapist; and, finally, provide **T**ime frames for achievement.

SMART Goals:
- **S**pecific descriptions of outcomes
- **M**easurable outcomes
- **A**ttainable outcomes based on a patient's unique characteristics, desired goals, and effectiveness of treatment
- **R**elevance and **T**ime frames primarily for the patient but also for the physical therapist

We encourage the use of SMART goals during patient care and believe that they can facilitate patient engagement and communication during health-care delivery. SMART goals are consistent with HOAC II and ICF and are designed to capture primarily the activity limitations and participation restrictions that led to the seeking of medical care for the patient's problems.

Now we need to prepare you for the upcoming chapters. Up to this point, we have presented broad conceptual principles, big-picture ideas that help to shape the health-care encounter and are directly related to outcome assessment. We must now dig a bit deeper into more specific and detailed concepts and principles that will serve as your foundation to an evidence-based approach to outcome assessment. We want to alert you to this shift in content delivery because we see the next several chapters as fundamentally different from, but strongly linked to, the material you have read to this point. We believe the upcoming content provides information that is essential to take full advantage of the rapidly burgeoning evidence on outcome assessment.

We made the case in Chapter 1 that the science of outcome assessment is akin, in substance and importance, to the recent evidence on diagnosis or treatment selection and that clinical practice can be enhanced by the application of this new science. We encourage you to be patient and to take your time while reading these next five chapters. Allow yourself some time to let this content sink in. The content may be challenging for some but we believe the time invested will be worth the effort. Mastering the material will permit you to be a critical consumer of the outcomes assessment literature and, we believe, will provide you with skills that will enhance your patients' care.

■ Reference List

1. Fairbank JC, Couper J, Davies JB, O'Brien JP. The Oswestry low back pain disability questionnaire. *Physiotherapy* 1980;66:271–3.

2. Hazard RG, Haugh LD, Green PA, Jones PL. Chronic low back pain: The relationship between patient satisfaction and pain, impairment, and disability outcomes. *Spine (Phila Pa 1976)* 1994;15;19:881–7.

3. Rantanen T, Guralnik JM, Izmirlian G, et al. Association of muscle strength with maximum walking speed in disabled older women. *Am J Phys Med Rehabil* 1998;77:299–305.

4. Buchner DM, Larson EB, Wagner EH, Koepsell TD, de Lateur BJ. Evidence for a non-linear relationship between leg strength and gait speed. *Age Ageing* 1996;25:386–91.

Chapter 4

How Confident Can I Be About the Outcome Measurement on My Patient?

Imagine taking a measurement on a patient and not having an idea about the extent of measurement error associated with the measurement. Would you be confident that the measurement was really meaningful and would you use it for making important clinical decisions? For example, let's say that your patient was being treated for a head injury and you were interested in quantifying the extent of spasticity in the patient's upper extremities. Would you be comfortable using a spasticity measure that your colleague recommended but that you had never used or read about? Without having a good idea of how much error is associated with a measurement, we do not know how confident we can be in a measured value or the clinical decisions based on the measurement.

What's Ahead

In this chapter, we provide a foundation for answering the question "How confident can I be about the score obtained for the outcome measure on my patient?" We show how the results from reliability studies can be used to provide estimates of measurement error. We cannot be confident that a measured value conveys useful information if we don't know the amount of error associated with the measurement. We begin our discussion by commenting on sources and types of measurement error. We then identify two frequently reported reliability coefficients and demonstrate how they are used to estimate measurement error. We conclude this chapter with an illustration of how the results from a reliability study can be applied to answer the question "How confident can I be about the outcome measurement on my patient?"

▶ The Concept Behind This Question

You'll notice that the title of this chapter (and subsequent chapters) is written in the form of a question. This chapter's question is based on the reality that error is unavoidable and present to some extent in all measurements no matter how much research and development has gone into constructing instruments. Sources of measurement error include the patient, examiner/ rater, environment, and measuring instrument. Table 4-1 provides examples of potential sources of measurement error applied to the measurement of knee flexion range of motion.

When we record a single value of an outcome measure in the medical record, we assume that the measurement error is sufficiently small as to not compromise the interpretation of the measurement and, more importantly, clinical decisions based on the measurement. In fact, the obtained value for a patient is just one of many possible values that could have been obtained at a single point in time. Figure 4-1 illustrates this concept. It represents 30 Timed-Up-and-Go (TUG) measurements obtained on a truly unchanged person (a person whose condition was unchanged and who did not receive interventions) over a 6-day period. Five measurements were performed each day and no systematic difference in measured values existed among days or trials within days. That is, the measured values were not influenced by the order in which they were obtained. The TUG test requires a person to rise from a standard armchair, walk at a safe and comfortable pace to a tape mark 3 m away, then return to a sitting position in the chair.[1] The test score is the time to complete the activity. The TUG is used to assess mobility and balance and it is regularly applied to diverse populations, including the elderly, persons with Parkinson disease, and persons with osteoarthritis. Typical estimates of test-retest reliability for the

Table 4-1 Potential Sources of Measurement Error Applied to Knee Flexion Range Measurements

Source		Example
Patient	Biologic variation	• On repeated knee flexion efforts the patient may provide different joint angles.
	Motivation	• The patient may try harder on some occasions compared to others.
Examiner/ Rater	Biologic variation	• Inherent variation in the examiner's senses.
	Instructions	• The instructions or amount of verbal encouragement may vary from one measurement session to the next.
	End digit preference	• The examiner may have a tendency to report specific numbers rather than the actual measured values (e.g., 0s and 5s).
	Expectation	• Knowing the previous value may influence the examiner's perception of the current measured value.
Environment	Disruptive environment	• This may distract the examiner or patient and result in an inaccurate reading.
	Inadequate lighting	• This may cause the examiner to read the goniometer incorrectly.
Measuring Instrument	Calibration/ scale	• Measuring range of motion to the closest 5 degrees because the goniometer is calibrated in 5-degree increments would yield different values compared to a goniometer calibrated in 1-degree increments.
	Defective instrument	• A goniometer with a "sloppy" pivot point would result in measurements with considerable variability.

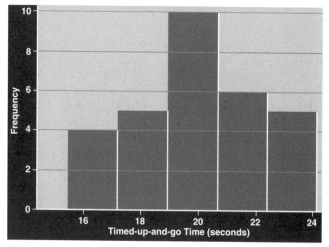

Figure 4-1 Histogram of 30 Timed-Up-and-Go Times on a Single Patient

TUG applied in the following contexts are 0.80 for persons with Parkinson disease,[2,3] 0.80 for a variety of inpatient orthopedic conditions,[4] and 0.75 for persons with osteoarthritis awaiting hip or knee replacement.[5] For the person whose measurements appear in Figure 4-1, the average TUG time was 20.0 seconds and the minimum and maximum times were 15.4 and 24.1 seconds, respectively.

In clinical practice we never know a patient's true value, but rather we infer it from the measured value. The relationship between measured values—often referred to as the observed score in the formal measurement literature—and true values is conveyed by the following expression:

$$\text{measured value} = \text{true value} + \text{error} \qquad (1)$$

where the error can take on positive or negative values. From this expression, we see that the smaller the measurement error, the closer the measured value is to the true value. Smaller measurement error translates into increased confidence in the measured value. Because clinical decisions are based on the interpretation of measured values rather than true values, the greater the confidence in the measured values, the greater the confidence in clinical decisions based on the measured values.

❚ Two Types of Measurement Error

Measurement error can be random or systematic. Random error is characterized by some measured values lying above the true value and other measured values falling below the true value. The data from our TUG example would suggest that in this patient the error in estimating the true value is random because no systematic differences were noted within or between days and the distribution of measured values approximates a bell-shaped or normal distribution with an approximately equal distribution of scores to the right and to the left of the mean value. If one were able to perform a large number of measurements on a truly unchanged patient, the average of the random errors would be zero, and the average of the measured values would equal the patient's true value. Applying this framework to our TUG example, the patient's average or true value is 20.0 seconds. When systematic error is present, the average error value will be greater than or less than zero, and the average of the measured values will also be greater than or less than the true value. For example, a slow-running stopwatch would give the appearance that persons performed the TUG faster than they actually did. When systematic error exists, it is superimposed on random error. Acknowledging that random and systematic errors can exist in the same measurement, the error term in Expression 1 can be expanded to read:

measured value = true value +
$$\text{(random error + systematic error)} \quad (2)$$

The Measurement Framework

Confidence in a measured value is characterized by the consistency or reproducibility of measured values for unchanged patients. Consistency is a requisite property to allow physical therapists to differentiate among patients who possess different amounts of the characteristic of interest. Differentiating among patients is essential when identifying patients' problems at the initial encounter and when determining whether a treatment goal has been met at follow-up. Reliability is the measurement property that quantifies the consistency of measured values and the ability of these values to differentiate among patients. At this point, it is important to acknowledge that tests and measures do not have reliabilities; measured scores do.[6] By focusing on measured scores, we are reminded that all measurements take place in a context. The context may be a set of patient characteristics, the condition of interest, or a specific time point in the natural or clinical history of patients with the condition of interest. Reliability studies usually consider random error. Also, it is important to remember that reliability studies do not address the extent to which a measure assesses what it is intended to measure: This measurement property is validity, and it is discussed in the next chapters.[7-10] The reliability version of Expression 1 is:

$$\text{measured value} = \text{true value} + \text{random error} \quad (3)$$

Applied in a reliability context, the true value is defined in a theoretical way as the average value that would have been obtained had an infinite number of measurements been applied to a truly unchanged patient. Reliability is important, not only because it provides the confidence in a measured value but also because it places an upper limit on validity. This is a very important clinical concept and one of the take-home messages of this chapter: A measure with low reliability is destined to have low validity and low clinical utility.

Reliability Coefficients: What Are They?

To this point, we have seen there are two conceptually important aspects of reliability, the ability to differentiate among patients and the consistency of measured values within a truly unchanged patient. It is therefore fitting that two methods for quantifying reliability are reported in the literature and of interest to physical therapists. The intraclass correlation coefficient (ICC) quantifies the ability of a measure's scores to differentiate among patients.

If you think of a goniometric measure of knee flexion, for example, we would like our goniometric measures to be able to differentiate between patients with mild and severe knee extensor contractures. If we couldn't differentiate between a patient with a mild and a patient with a severe contracture, we would have to question whether the goniometric measure is worthwhile in the first place.

The ICC is a unitless quantity that can take values from 0 to 1 (it is calculated as the true score variance divided by the observed score variance). Larger values represent greater reliability. Because the ICC is unitless, it is referred to as a "relative" reliability coefficient. In contrast, the standard error of measurement (SEM)* quantifies the consistency of measured values in the same units as the original measurement. Smaller SEMs represent greater consistency and smaller measurement errors. The SEM is termed an "absolute" reliability coefficient because it quantifies measurement error in the same units as the original measurement. For a measure to be clinically useful in a specific context, it must have a sufficiently high ICC and a sufficiently low SEM. What do a sufficiently high ICC and a sufficiently low SEM really mean? It depends on the measurement and on the clinical decision you are considering. We illustrate this concept later in this chapter.

Rationale for Reliability Studies

Because physical therapists' decisions are based on measured or observed values rather than true values, knowing the reliability of a measurement is essential when forming an opinion about the confidence in a clinical decision based on a measurement. In clinical practice, it is impractical to estimate measurement error by obtaining a large number of measurements on a truly unchanged patient as was done with our TUG example. Typically, in clinical practice, a single measurement or several measurements are performed at a single patient encounter. The difficulty from an interpretive perspective is that measurement

---

* Do not confuse the standard error of measurement with the standard error of the mean.

error is at play and the obtained value could lie close to a patient's true value (e.g., 19.6 seconds for our TUG example) or at some distance from a patient's true value (e.g., 24.1 seconds). Accordingly, it is necessary for a physical therapist to know the typical amount of error associated with a truly unchanged patient's response. So where, then, does an estimate of measurement error or variability come from if it is not feasible to obtain a large number of measurements on a single patient? The answer to this question is that this estimate comes from a test-retest reliability study.

Rather than obtaining many measurements on a single patient, a test-retest reliability study obtains two or more measurements on each of many stable patients (those who should not have changed because of a short time interval and who had no intervening treatment) with the condition of interest. Each patient contributes an estimate of variability (i.e., the difference between test and retest values) that is combined into a single estimate of measurement error in the units of interest. This error estimate is known as the SEM. There are several advantages to this approach. First, it is feasible to obtain two measurements on many patients rather than submitting a single patient to many measurements. Second, it is possible to obtain estimates of the measure's ability to differentiate among patients (ICC), as well as the measurement error in the same units as the original measurement (SEM). Third, by sampling many patients, one is able to generalize the results to a larger group of patients with characteristics similar to those patients taking part in the reliability study.

What to Look for When Reviewing a Reliability Study

Making a judgment about a patient's progress typically involves a comparison between the current and previous assessments' values for the outcome of interest. Because these measurements are obtained on different occasions, a test-retest reliability study design offers the most informative approach to determining relative (ICC) and absolute (SEM) reliability coefficients. To have confidence in the results of a test-retest reliability study it is essential that no true change in patients occurs between test and retest. Ideally, authors should comment on this point;

however, if they do not, readers could compare the outcome measure's mean test and retest values. Although, due to sampling variability, one would not expect these means to be identical, a substantial difference in either a positive or negative direction would provide evidence that patients changed over the course of the reliability study. A second important requirement for the results to be useful is that the distribution of difference scores between test and retest are consistent with a normal distribution. A significant deviation from a normal distribution suggests the measurement error may not be random. Once again, the author should state this and there is little readers can do to check this assumption in the absence of such a statement.

Our final comment is more of a warning: Don't be impressed by authors' proclamations that the results show the measure is reliable. Summary statements of many reliable studies often conclude that a test or measure is reliable. There are two problems with such a statement. First, reliability is not an all-or-none property—reliability exists to a degree. Second, reliability is not a property of a measure, but rather of a measure's scores.[6] The second point reminds us that measurements take place in a context and that the reliability of a measure in one context may well differ from the reliability of the same measure in a different context. For example, the reliability of the 6-minute walk test may be different for persons with respiratory problems compared to persons with osteoarthritis at the hip.

Can I Calculate the SEM If It Has Not Been Reported?

Often researchers have reported ICCs but not SEMs. This practice is unfortunate because the SEM provides an indication of measurement error in units familiar to physical therapists. However, in many instances investigators have supplied sufficient information to allow readers to calculate the SEM. We present the following vignette to show three essentially equivalent methods of calculating the SEM that draw on different information.[11] Before proceeding, we wish to stress that it is not a requirement that readers know how to perform an analysis of variance (ANOVA) or calculate a standard deviation; all that is necessary is that readers can use the information if it is provided.

In this hypothetical example, an investigator performed a test-retest reliability study on 60 patients with Parkinson disease. Table 4-2 provides a representation of the data along with the means and standard deviations for the two occasions and the difference between occasions. We see that mean values for test and retest are essentially equal. Table 4-3 displays the analysis of variance table. Figure 4-2 shows that the distribution of difference scores between test and retest is consistent with a normal distribution.

Table 4-2 Test, Retest, and Differences in TUG Time Values

Patient	Test	Retest	Difference Between Test-Retest
1	14.28	15.50	−1.22
2	19.08	18.25	0.83
3	22.67	21.61	1.06
.	.	.	.
.	.	.	.
.	.	.	.
58	14.34	16.42	−2.08
59	14.75	18.25	−3.50
60	17.73	15.06	2.67
Mean	17.95	17.80	0.15
SD	2.35	2.12	1.56

Table 4-3 Analysis of Variance Table with Variance Components

Source	Degrees of Freedom	Sum of Squares	Mean Squares	Variance Components
Patient	59	518.9	8.8	3.8
Error	60	72.8	1.2	1.2
Total	119	591.9		5.0

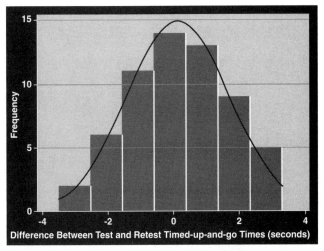

Figure 4-2 Distribution of TUG Time Differences Between Test and Retest Measurements for 60 Truly Unchanged Patients

Using the information provided in Tables 4-2 and 4-3, the SEM can be calculated as follows:

Method 1: Uses the Error Variance or Mean Square Error Term for the ANOVA Table

$$SEM = \sqrt{\text{error variance}}$$
$$SEM = \sqrt{1.2}$$
$$SEM = 1.1 \text{ seconds}$$

Method 2: Uses the Pooled Occasion Standard Deviation and ICC

$$SEM = \text{pooled occasion standard deviation}\sqrt{1-ICC}$$
$$SEM = \sqrt{(2.35^2 + 2.12^2)/2} \times \sqrt{1-0.76}$$
$$SEM = 1.1 \text{ seconds}$$

Method 3:   Uses the Standard Deviation of Difference
Scores Between Test and Retest

$$SEM = \frac{standard\ deviation\ of\ test\text{-}retest\ difference}{\sqrt{2}}$$

$$SEM = \frac{1.56}{\sqrt{2}}$$

$$SEM = 1.1\ seconds$$

For each analysis the SEM was calculated to be 1.1 seconds.
Although multiple measurements per patient are necessary to
estimate the ICC and SEM, as calculated and presented in
many articles, they represent the theoretical reliability for a
single measurement.

▶ Translating Reliability Coefficients into Clinically Useful Information

In the previous example the ICC was 0.76 and the SEM was
1.1 seconds. However, two questions frequently asked are:
(1) "To be clinically useful, how high must the ICC be?" and
(2) "How do I use the SEM?" There is no one answer that satis-
fies the first question; however, authorities do agree on the following guidelines:

1. for the ICC, the larger the better.
2. greater levels of reliability are required when making
   decisions concerning individuals compared to groups.
3. the reliability of the measure of interest should be
   comparable to, or better than, those of other measures
   intended for the same purpose when applied in a similar
   context.

We have mentioned previously that when physical therapists
record a single measured value in the medical record they are
assuming the measurement error is sufficiently small to justify
use of the instrument. They have equated the measured value
with the true value. However, rather than thinking that a

patient's measured value equals the true value, it is more appropriate to think of the measured value as representing an estimate of the true value. The extent to which one can have confidence that the measured value provides a reasonable estimate of the true value can be determined by constructing a confidence interval that is likely to contain a patient's true value. This is done by multiplying the SEM by the z-value (i.e., a standardized value obtained from a standard normal table located in the appendices of most statistical textbooks) for the confidence level of interest. One SEM is equal to a 68% confidence interval; 1.65 SEMs is equal to a 90% confidence interval; and 1.96 SEMs is equal to a 95% confidence interval. So if a patient's measured TUG time were 20.0 seconds, the 90% confidence interval would be from 18.2 to 21.8 seconds (i.e., 20 ± [1.1 seconds × 1.65]). We would therefore be 90% confident that the patient's "true" score was somewhere between 18.2 and 21.8 seconds. There is more on how this single-score estimate can be used to help interpret the meaningfulness of change scores in Chapter 6.

The Bottom Line

Useful information can be obtained from methodologically sound test-retest reliability studies provided they consist of a relevant patient sample. Acceptable levels of relative and absolute reliability coefficients are necessary, but insufficient, to support the validity of a measure.

A Clinical Example **What the Researcher Did**

This example is based on a test-retest reliability study reported by Huang et al.[3] These researchers investigated the test-retest reliability of the TUG applied to 72 patients with Parkinson disease. The study sample was drawn from patients attending a specialty clinic for movement disorders at a university hospital. Patients fulfilling the eligibility criteria were assessed on two occasions approximately 2 weeks apart. Huang et al reported a test-retest ICC of 0.80. The mean (SD) TUG times for the test and retest assessments were 11.8 (2.9) and 11.8 (3.4) seconds, respectively. The mean (SD) difference was 0 (2.0) seconds. Information provided by these authors allows the calculation of the SEM using Methods 2 and 3 described previously.

Method 2 Calculation of the SEM

SEM = pooled occasion standard deviation$\sqrt{1-R}$

SEM = $\sqrt{(2.9^2 + 3.4^2)/2} \times \sqrt{1-0.80}$

SEM = 1.4 seconds

Method 3 Calculation of the SEM

$$SEM = \frac{\text{standard deviation of test-retest difference}}{\sqrt{2}}$$

$$SEM = \frac{2.0}{\sqrt{2}}$$

SEM = 1.4 seconds

How the Physical Therapist Applied the Information

Being familiar with the study of Huang et al, a physical therapist applied the information to Mr. Park, a patient with characteristics similar to those participating in the Huang et al study. Mr. Park's TUG time was 12.2 seconds. Applying a 90% confidence level, the physical therapist interprets Mr. Park's true value to be 12.2 ± 2.3 seconds and records the following in the medical record: TUG time 12.2 (90% CI: 9.9, 14.5).

A Bit More: Reducing Measurement Error by Averaging Measured Values

Suppose that Mr. Park's physical therapist believed that the error or confidence interval for the TUG time was too large. One way to improve the reliability of a measured value is to optimize the approach used (i.e., procedural components) to acquire the measurement. Examples of procedural components are listed in Table 4-1. One approach for increasing reliability is to obtain multiple measurements and average their results. Once again, a key assumption is that a patient's true value has not changed between occasions. Averaging multiple measured values affects the SEM by a factor equal to the square root of the number of measurements contributing to the average. For example, the SEM for the average of two measurements is calculated as follows:

$$\text{Averaged SEM} = \frac{\text{SEM}}{\sqrt{\text{number of measurements}}}$$

$$\text{Averaged SEM} = \frac{1.4}{\sqrt{2}}$$

$$\text{Averaged SEM} = 0.99 \text{ seconds}$$

Had the physical therapist in the above example obtained two measurements on Mr. Park and recorded the average value, the 90% confidence interval on the average value would have been ±1.6 seconds (10.6 to 13.8 seconds) rather than ±2.3 seconds (9.9 to 14.5 seconds) obtained for a single measurement.

Chapter Summary

- Sources of measurement error include the patient, examiner, environment, and measuring instrument.
- Measurement error can be random and systemic.
- Reliability considers random error only.
- There are two aspects to reliability: (1) the consistency of measured values and (2) the ability of the measure to differentiate among patients.
- Applied in a clinical context, absolute reliability quantifies the consistency of measured values and expresses measurement error in the same units as the original measurement.
- Applied in a clinical context, relative reliability quantifies the ability of a measure to differentiate among patients.
- Information from reliability studies can be used to express the confidence in a measured value.
- The greater the confidence in a measured value, the greater the confidence in clinical decisions based on the measured value.
- Reliability is a necessary but insufficient requirement when determining the ability of a measure to assess what it is intended to measure (validity).

▪ Reference List

1. Podsiadlo D, Richardson S. The timed "Up & Go": A test of basic functional mobility for frail elderly persons. *J Am Geriatr Soc* 1991;39: 142–8.

2. Steffen T, Seney M. Test-retest reliability and minimal detectable change on balance and ambulation tests, the 36-item short-form health survey, and the unified Parkinson disease rating scale in people with parkinsonism. *Phys Ther* 2008;88:733–46.

3. Huang SL, Hsieh CL, Wu RM, Tai CH, Lin CH, Lu WS. Minimal detectable change of the timed "up & go" test and the dynamic gait index in people with Parkinson disease. *Phys Ther* 2011;91:114–21.

4. Yeung TS, Wessel J, Stratford PW, MacDermid JC. The timed up and go test for use on an inpatient orthopaedic rehabilitation ward. *J Orthop Sports Phys Ther* 2008;38:410–7.

5. Kennedy DM, Stratford PW, Wessel J, Gollish JD, Penney D. Assessing stability and change of four performance measures: A longitudinal study evaluating outcome following total hip and knee arthroplasty. *BMC Musculoskelet Disord* 2005;6:3.

6. Messick S. Validity. In: Linn RL, editor. *Educational Measurement*, 3rd ed. Phoenix, AZ: ORYZ Press;1993: p. 14.

7. Rothstein JM. *Measurement and Clinical Practice: Theory and Application. Measurement in Physical Therapy.* New York: Churchill Livingstone;1985.

8. McDowell I, Newell C. Measuring Health: A guide to Rating Scales and Questionnaires, 2nd ed. New York: Oxford University Press;1996.

9. Nunnally JC. *Psychometric Theory.* Toronto: McGraw-Hill;1978.

10. Feldt LS, Brennan RL. Reliability. In: Linn RL, editor. *Educational Measurement.* Phoenix, AZ: Oryx Press;1993.

11. Stratford PW. Getting more from the literature: Estimating the standard error of measurement from reliability studies. *Physiother Can* 2004;56: 27–30.

Chapter 5

What Does This Outcome Measurement Really Mean?

▪ *What would it take for you to add a test or measure to a patient's assessment or to replace a measure you are currently using? When faced with this question, one of our colleagues answered this way: "To take the extra time and effort required to administer and score a new measure, it must provide additional clinically useful information and lead to more confident decisions than obtained from my current assessment methods."*

There are three important points raised in this statement. One is that the measure must provide a greater amount of useful information than is currently available. The second point introduces the notion of confidence. In mentioning confidence, this physical therapist is acknowledging that the information obtained from measures contains error and that some measures will be better than others for a given purpose. The final concept considers the reality of time. In a busy practice, one must efficiently maximize information and confidence in clinical decisions.

What's Ahead

The previous chapter dealt with random error and its application in determining the confidence in a measured value. It did not consider the degree to which the measure was assessing the characteristic of interest. In this chapter, we build on the previous one by considering the extent to which valid inferences can be drawn from a measure's values. Historically, validity focused on the integrity of a measure and it was not uncommon to see validity referred to as a property of a measure. For example, "the 6-minute walk test has a high level of validity." Subsequently, it was realized that validity is not a property of a measure, but rather of a measure's scores or values.[1] This distinction is important because it directs one's attention to the context in which measurements are obtained. The context includes patient characteristics, clinical setting, and conditions of measurement. When considering validity today, our attention is no longer restricted to validity coefficients and measured values, but rather the emphasis is now on the inferences we can confidently draw from the measured values.[2] In other words, "What does this outcome measurement really mean?" In this chapter, we answer this question by responding to two inextricably linked questions:

1. To what extent does a measure assess what it is intended to measure within a declared context?
2. What is the interpretation of a measured value?

The first question considers traditional validation procedures and the latter question addresses interpretability. Interpretability comments on the extent to which qualitative meaning can be assigned to quantitative values.[3]

▶ Part 1: To What Extent Does the Measure Assess What It Is Intended to Measure?

The Concept Behind This Question

Applied in a reliability context, the term *true value* represents the average of a conceptually infinite number of measurements when only random error is at play. As such, the reliability "true value" does not reflect the extent to which a measure assesses what it is intended to measure. Although reliability is a necessary requirement, it alone does not ensure a measure's usefulness. *Validity* is the term used to describe the extent to which correct inferences can be made about the characteristic of interest. Thus, in addition to random error, validity also considers systematic error. Within a validity context, the relationship between the measured and true values can be expressed as follows:

measured value = true value + random error + systematic error

This relationship shows that validity increases as random and systematic errors decrease. Finally, like reliability, validity is not an all-or-none measurement property, but rather it exists to a degree along a continuum.

The Measurement Framework

The essence of validation studies is the forming and testing of hypotheses concerning what a measure should detect on a specific sample.[4] For some outcomes of interest to physical therapists, criterion standards exist (e.g., range of motion, strength) and, therefore, validity is a straightforward comparison of the criterion's values with those of the outcome measure. However for many important outcomes, there are no criterion standards (e.g., pain, functional status, health-related quality of life), so determining the extent of validity for these types of measures is more challenging.

Types of Validity

Content validity examines the extent to which a measure adequately samples items or activities from the domain of interest. In this context, content validity applies most directly to self-report or performance-based measures that attempt to capture a multitude of dimensions or constructs. For example, in considering lower extremity functional status one would expect to see items on walking on level ground, transferring (e.g., chair to standing, into the bathtub, etc.), going up and down stairs, squatting, and running—to name a few. There is no formal statistical analysis to assess content validity; rather, it is evaluated by gaining consensus from an expert panel of stakeholders that the items composing the measure are relevant and representative of the domain of interest.

Construct validity exists to the extent that a measure's values provide results consistent with theories concerning the patient sample of interest and the characteristic being tested. Construct validation of a measure typically applies to one or more of the following three approaches. Convergent construct validation is based on the idea that measures believed to be assessing the same characteristic should correlate highly. For example, Pua et al reported a correlation of 0.78 between Lower Extremity Functional Scale (LEFS) values (Fig. 5-1) and Western Ontario and McMaster Universities Osteoarthritis Index physical function (WOMAC-PF) subscale values.[5] Known group construct validation applies the theory that identifiable groups have different levels of the characteristic of interest. For example, investigators theorized that lower LEFS values would be obtained for patients who were post hip or knee arthroplasty and required home care compared to those patients not requiring home care.[6] A comparison of the group means supported the LEFS' ability to distinguish between these groups of patients: LEFS mean value home care = 15.2; LEFS mean not requiring home care = 23.7.[6]

Discriminant construct validation is based on the notion that measures intended to assess the same characteristic should correlate more highly than measures intended to assess different characteristics. For example, Pua et al reported a correlation of 0.75 between the LEFS and SF-36 physical function subscale compared to a correlation of 0.60 between the LEFS and SF-36 pain subscale.[5]

Criterion validity exists to the extent that a measure provides results consistent with a gold standard. Criterion validation studies compare a measure's values with those of a gold or criterion standard. For example, Bohannon applied a criterion validation design to estimate the validity of manual muscle testing applied to the assessment of knee extensor strength.[7] Using hand-held dynamometry as the criterion standard, a Spearman's correlation of 0.77 was obtained.

Cross-sectional and Longitudinal Validity

Two essential properties of outcome measures are their ability to discriminate among patients at a point in time and to detect

LOWER EXTREMITY FUNCTIONAL SCALE

We are interested in knowing whether you are having any difficulty at all with the activities listed below **because of your lower limb** problem for which you are currently seeking attention.

Please provide an answer for each activity. Today, **do you** or **would you** have any difficulty at all with: (Circle one number on each line)

ACTIVITIES	Extreme Difficulty or Unable to Perform Activity	Quite a bit of Difficulty	Moderate Difficulty	A Little bit of Difficulty	No Difficulty
a. Any of your usual work, housework, or school activities	0	1	2	3	4
b. Your usual hobbies, or recreational or sporting activities	0	1	2	3	4
c. Getting into or out of the bath	0	1	2	3	4
d. Walking between rooms	0	1	2	3	4
e. Putting on your shoes or socks	0	1	2	3	4
f. Squatting	0	1	2	3	4
g. Lifting an object, like a bag of groceries, from the floor	0	1	2	3	4
h. Performing light activities around your home	0	1	2	3	4
i. Performing heavy activities around your home	0	1	2	3	4
j. Getting into or out of a car	0	1	2	3	1
k. Walking 2 blocks	0	1	2	3	1
l. Walking a mile	0	1	2	3	4
m. Going up or down 10 stairs (about 1 flight)	0	1	2	3	4
n. Standing for 1 hour	0	1	2	3	4
o. Sitting for 1 hour	0	1	2	3	4
p. Running on even ground	0	1	2	3	4
q. Running on uneven ground	0	1	2	3	4
r. Making sharp turns while running fast	0	1	2	3	4
s. Hopping	0	1	2	3	4
t. Rolling over in bed	0	1	2	3	4
Column totals:					

©1996 JM Binkley, reprinted w/permission   Score: _____ /80

Figure 5-1 Lower Extremity Functional Scale

change over time. Cross-sectional validity assesses the extent to which a measure provides a valid representation of the characteristic of interest at a point in time. Longitudinal validity investigates the extent to which a measure detects valid change over time. Similar analyses are applied to cross-sectional and longitudinal validation studies. The only difference is that cross-sectional analyses consider a single value obtained at a point in time, whereas longitudinal studies assess a change score (i.e., the difference between the previous and current assessments' values). In this chapter, our focus is on cross-sectional validity. In Chapter 6 we discuss longitudinal validation methods.

Validity Coefficients

Although a variety of validity coefficients exist, correlation coefficients and between-group test statistics are predominantly applied to outcome measure validation studies. When evaluating convergent construct validity or criterion validity, Pearson's correlation coefficient is used when the data are consistent with a normal distribution and have interval scale properties; otherwise, distribution-free tests such as Spearman's rank order correlation coefficient are applied.[8] When assessing known group construct validity, t-tests and analysis of variance are used when the data are consistent with a normal distribution and have interval scale properties. If data do not possess these properties, Wilcoxon's rank sum and Kruskal-Wallis' distribution-free tests are typically performed.[8]

A Clinical Example   **What the Researcher Did**

In this hypothetical example, an investigator was interested in determining the extent to which a region-specific self-report measure of lower extremity functional status, the Lower Extremity Functional Scale (LEFS), was valid when applied to patients with osteoarthritis of the knee who were awaiting total knee joint arthroplasty (TKA). The LEFS consists of 20 items, each of which is scored on a 0- to 4-point scale.[9] Higher LEFS scores represent higher levels of lower extremity functional status. Because no gold standard for lower extremity functional status exists, the investigator applied convergent, discriminant, and known group construct validation methods. The convergent construct validation component theorized that LEFS scores would display a high correlation (Pearson $|r| > 0.80$) with Western Ontario and McMaster Universities Osteoarthritis Index physical function subscale scores (WOMAC-PF). The WOMAC-PF (Likert version 3.1) contains 17 items, each of which is scored on a 5-point scale.[10] Total WOMAC-PF scores can vary from 0 to 68, with lower scores representing higher levels of functional status. The discriminant construct validation component theorized that LEFS scores would display a higher correlation with WOMAC-PF scores than with WOMAC pain (WOMAC-PN) scores. Based on previous work, the known group construct validation component theorized that women awaiting total joint arthroplasty would display greater disability and, therefore, lower LEFS scores than men. A convenience sample of 44 women and 40 men fulfilling the eligibility criteria participated in the study. Patients were administered the LEFS and WOMAC at the same occasion approximately 2 weeks prior to TKA.

To evaluate whether the correlation between the LEFS and WOMAC-PF exceeded 0.80, Pearson's correlation coefficient was calculated and tested against the null value of 0.80.[8] To determine whether the correlation between the LEFS and WOMAC-PF was greater than between the LEFS and WOMAC-PN, Pearson's correlation coefficients were calculated and compared using Meng's test for dependent data applied.[11] To evaluate whether women displayed more disability than men, a t-test for independent sample means was applied.[8]

Figure 5-2 shows the scatterplot of WOMAC-PF and LEFS data. Convergent construct validity was supported to the extent that the absolute correlation ($|r|$) between the measures' scores was 0.86, and this value statistically exceeded 0.80 ($p = 0.040$).

Discriminant construct validity was supported to the extent that the absolute correlation between LEFS and WOMAC-PN scores was 0.68, which was significantly lower ($p < 0.001$) than the correlation of 0.86 between LEFS and WOMAC-PF scores. Known group construct validity was supported to the extent that the mean (SD) women's LEFS score of 28.7 (11.1) was significantly less ($p = 0.002$) than the mean men's LEFS score of 36.5 (12.9).

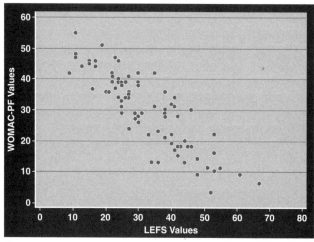

Figure 5-2 Scatterplot of WOMAC-PF and LEFS Scores

How Physical Therapists Applied the Information

A group of physical therapists already using the LEFS to assess patients' post-ankle sprain were interested in whether it could also be applied with confidence to patients with OA of the knee awaiting TKA. The physical therapists interpreted the results from the preceding study as providing support for the validity and clinical use of LEFS on patients with osteoarthritis awaiting TKA. This hypothetical study did not provide estimates of how to interpret LEFS scores, but it did support the theoretical validity of the LEFS on patients scheduled for knee arthroplasty. In other words, the hypothetical study provided some but not all of the information required to feel confident about using the measure for daily practice decisions.

▶ Part 2: What Is the Interpretation of the Measured Value?

Interpretability is defined as the ability to assign qualitative meaning to quantitative scores.[3] Stated another way, interpretability considers the extent to which unitless scores, such as those obtained with the LEFS, can be translated into meaningful representations of the characteristic of interest.

The Concept Behind the Interpretability Question

One decision made at a patient's initial assessment is whether a measured value provides evidence of a deficiency or limitation for the measurement characteristic of interest (e.g., range of motion, functional status, work status). To effectively make this decision, a physical therapist must be able to assign meaning to the measured value. For some measures, interpreting a value is done effortlessly; for other measures a value's meaning is less obvious.

For example, consider a person who has a 2-week post-TKA passive knee flexion of 86° and a LEFS score of 16. Understanding the meaning of 86° of knee flexion is done effortlessly. Without much thought, it is likely that a vivid picture of a knee flexed to 86° pops into your head. You may also quickly develop an interpretation of the meaning of this measure. For example, based on other literature that you have read, you confidently judge that the patient will likely have difficulty negotiating stairs normally with only 86° of knee flexion. Given that the patient lives in a two-story home, you have very quickly assigned a high level of importance to this finding. A greater challenge is to assign meaning to relatively new self-report measures' values. For example, what level of lower extremity functional status does a LEFS score of 16 represent? The interpretation of the LEFS score is not as intuitive as the range-of-motion value. Nor is there as much evidence published to guide the interpretation of a self-report functional status measure as compared to a range-of-motion measurement, for example. In this section we illustrate an approach for assigning qualitative meaning to quantitative scores of measurements that may not have a high level of intuitive meaning.

Interpretation of Measures' Scores That Are Not Highly Intuitive

The past three decades have seen a proliferation of multi-item self-report measures. These measures assess many important outcomes of interest to physical therapists. Although the concepts being assessed (e.g., pain, functional status, emotional well-being) are self-evident, the scores produced by the measures often lack meaning, particularly when a measure is relatively new. In this section, we illustrate one approach for assigning meaning to such measures' scores. Our example considers the interpretation of a LEFS score of 16.

At first glance, it would seem quite simple to interpret the meaning of a LEFS value or that of any other multi-item health status measure: We would form an impression by looking at the item responses endorsed by a patient. For example, to gain an impression of a patient's ability to cope with heavy activities around the house, we would simply look at the patient's response to this item. Unfortunately, translating responses on a self-report functional status measure into a meaningful representation of a patient's functional status is not this easy. The reason is that multi-item measures are typically validated at the total score level, or in the case of indexes with multiple domains (e.g., physical function, social function, pain, mental health), at the subscale level. The error associated with a single item value is usually too large to be interpreted with confidence. For this reason, the total score value must be translated into a meaningful representation of a patient's functional status level. To accomplish this, one works backwards from the total score to form an impression of the functional status for a typical person presenting with the total score value of interest. An item difficulty map (Table 5-1) provides an effective and efficient method of presenting this information.[12] Referring to Table 5-1, we see that a typical person with a LEFS score of 16— remember the 90% confidence interval for a LEFS value is ±6

Table 5-1	Item Difficulty Map for the LEFS[12]			
LEFS Score	**Quite a Bit of Difficulty**	**Moderate Difficulty**	**A Little Bit of Difficulty**	**No Difficulty**
80				
75				run uneven sharp turns run even
70				heavy activities
65			run uneven sharp turns	walk 1-mile stairs
60			run even walk 1-mile heavy activities	walk 2-blocks light activities in/out bath
55		run even	stairs	
50				
45		walk 1-mile heavy activities	walk 2-blocks light activities in/out bath	
40		stairs walk 2-blocks		
35				
30		in/out bath light activities	walk between rooms	
25	heavy activities stairs walk 2-blocks			
20	in/out bath light activities	walk between rooms		
15				
10	walk between rooms			
5				
0				

points—would have quite a bit of difficulty with light activities around the home, getting into and out of the bath, and perhaps walking between rooms. Accordingly, our impression of a specific patient with a LEFS value of 16 is shaped by the activity-difficulty relationship of a typical patient with this LEFS value, rather than the response pattern for the specific patient of interest.

Chapter Summary

- The extent to which valid influences can be drawn from a measure's value is dependent on the ability of a measure to assess what it is intended to measure and the extent to which a clinically useful interpretation can be assigned to a measured value.
- Validation studies examine the extent to which measures assess what they are intended to measure within a declared context.
- The essence of validation studies is the forming and testing of hypotheses concerning what the measure should detect on a specific sample.
- Types of validity frequently encountered in the literature include content, construct, and criterion validity.
- Construct validity is often subdivided into three categories: convergent, known group, and discriminant.
- Interpretability comments on the extent to which qualitative meaning can be assigned to quantitative values.
- Measures validated at the total score or subscale level cannot be interpreted with confidence at the item level.

■ Reference List

1. Messick S. Validity. In: Linn RL, editor. *Educational Measurement*, 3rd ed. Phoenix, AZ: ORYZ Press;1993: p. 14.

2. Landy FJ. Stamp collecting versus science: Validation as hypothesis testing. *Am Psychol* 1986;41:1183–92.

3. Mokkink LB, Terwee CB, Patrick DL, Alonso J, Stratford PW, Knol DL, et al. The COSMIN study reached international consensus on taxonomy, terminology, and definitions of measurement properties for

health-related patient-reported outcomes. *J Clin Epidemiol* 2010;63: 737–45.

4. Lawshe CH. Inferences from personnel tests and their validity. *J Appl Psychol* 1985;70:237–8.

5. Pua YH, Cowan SM, Wrigley TV, Bennell KL. The Lower Extremity Functional Scale could be an alternative to the Western Ontario and McMaster Universities Osteoarthritis Index physical function scale. *J Clin Epidemiol* 2009;62:1103–11.

6. Stratford PW, Binkley JM, Watson J, Heath-Jones T. Validation of the LEFS on patients with total joint arthroplasty. *Physiother Can* 2000;52: 97–105, 10.

7. Bohannon RW. Measuring knee extensor muscle strength. *Am J Phys Med Rehabil* 2001;80:13–8.

8. Daniel WW. *Biostatistics a Foundation for Analysis in the Health Sciences*, 9th ed. Hoboken, NJ: Wiley;2009.

9. Binkley JM, Stratford PW, Lott SA, Riddle DL. The Lower Extremity Functional Scale (LEFS): Scale development, measurement, properties, and clinical application. The North American Orthopaedic Rehabilitation Research Network. *Phys Ther* 1999;79:371–83.

10. Bellamy N. *WOMAC Osteoarthritis Index User Guide IV*. Queensland, Australia: University of Queensland; 2000.

11. Meng X, Rosenthal R, Rubin DB. Comparing correlated correlation coefficients. *Psychol Bull* 1992;111:172–5.

12. Stratford PW, Hart DL, Binkley JM, Kennedy DM, Alcock GK, Hanna SE. Interpreting Lower Extremity Functional Status Scores. *Physiother Can* 2005;57:154–62.

Chapter 6

What Does a Change in the Outcome Measurement Indicate?

■ Have you ever reassessed a patient by repeating measurements and wondered whether the change (either improvement or worsening) that may have occurred indicated real and important change or whether it was simply measurement error? More than likely, the smaller this change, the more you questioned whether it was real or important. Well, if you answered yes to the question, we are not surprised. Judging change is one of the most common dilemmas faced by physical therapists with practically every patient at some point during the plan of care. In Chapter 1 we stated, "The conscientious and judicious assessment of patients' outcomes is a complex clinical skill, much like patient assessment and treatment selection and delivery, and requires a conceptual framework and a specific body of knowledge." Perhaps nowhere is the complexity of outcome assessment more evident than in understanding the interpretation of change scores. Key to this issue is the interpretation of threshold values of change supplied in different research papers and secondarily in many textbooks.

When deciding whether a patient has improved (or worsened), a physical therapist judges whether the difference between current and previous assessments' values meets a predetermined threshold value, and this impression regarding whether change has occurred or not is recorded in the medical record. Historically, decisions concerning a patient's change status were guided by clinical experience alone. Today, *study-based threshold values for many measures are available to augment clinical experience. Ideally, study-based estimates of change complement clinical experience by providing not only an evidence-based threshold value but also a representation of the confidence a physical therapist can have in making the correct decision when applying the threshold value.*

Figure 6-1 introduces the possible consequences faced by a physical therapist when deciding whether a patient has or has not improved. This figure reminds us that not all patients with change scores meeting the reported threshold value will be truly improved. Neither will all patients with change scores less than the threshold value be unimproved. Physical therapists can be confident in their decisions to the extent that the threshold value accurately classifies the change status of patients. For an outcome measure to be clinically useful, a physical therapist must know the threshold value for change and be confident that applying this value provides a good chance of correctly labeling a patient's true change status.

What's Ahead

In this chapter we describe three popular methods used by researchers to estimate threshold change values for individual patients. We also explain the interpretation of these estimates and

		True Change Status	
		Improved	Unimproved
Physical Therapist's Interpretation of Change Score	Threshold change value met	Correctly labeled improved	Incorrectly labeled improved
	Threshold change value not met	Incorrectly labeled unimproved	Correctly labeled unimproved

Figure 6-1 Possible Results When Interpreting a Patient's Change Score

compare the information offered by each method to the information required by physical therapists when making decisions about the change status of patients. In addition, we alert readers to three other critical points when considering important change. The first is that the magnitude of a clinically important change for an individual patient is much greater than the clinically important difference between two groups of patients, such as comparisons done in clinical trials.[1,2] The second point acknowledges that the value for a clinically important change will likely be influenced by the cost, inconvenience, and potential benefits and harms associated with a specific intervention.[3–5] The final point is that the threshold value for an important change is likely to vary depending on a patient's previous assessment's value.[1,6–10] It seems the worse off a patient is, the greater the change necessary to be considered important.

Abbreviations in this Chapter

DTM	Diagnostic Test Methodology
ROC	Receiver Operating Characteristic Curve
AUC	Area Under the Curve
MDC	Minimal Detectable Change
RCI	Reliability Change Index
PIM	Percentile Improvement Method
MCID	Minimal Clinically Important Difference
MCII	Minimal Clinically Important Improvement

The Concept Behind the Question: What Does a Change in the Outcome Measurement Indicate?

When making a decision about a patient's change status a physical therapist compares the current and previous assessments' values. If the change meets a preconceived threshold value, a patient is labeled as having changed. However, in actuality a patient's true change status remains unknown. Referring back to Figure 6-1, we see that physical therapists arrive at their decisions by working horizontally in the table. A test is applied; it is interpreted; and a patient's change status is declared without knowing the truth. In contrast, researchers establish threshold values by referencing patients' change scores to their true change status as determined by a reference or gold standard. Referring to Figure 6-1, we see that researchers work vertically in this table: The true change status is known and it is used to determine the threshold value that best discriminates between improved and unimproved patients. This distinction matters because we will learn that expressions of "vertical" accuracy, using Figure 6-1 as a reference, do not provide direct interpretations of "horizontal" accuracy. Stated another way, patients correctly identified by the threshold value as being improved based on the researcher's perspective differ from patients correctly identified by the threshold value as improved based on the physical therapist's perspective. We develop this concept further as we describe and compare three popular methods used to estimate threshold change values.

▶ Diagnostic Test Method of Estimating Threshold Value for Change

Diagnostic test methodology (DTM) is an application of signal detection theory that was originally developed during World War Two to optimize the signal-to-noise ratio in applications such as radar and sonar.[11] DTM has a long history of use in the medical field to assess the accuracy of tests and measures where the goal is to discriminate between two groups (e.g., condition present or absent). Over two decades ago, Deyo and Centor recognized that DTM provides an ideal method for identifying threshold change values.[12] Applied in this context the goal is to diagnose a patient's change status. Although DTM can be applied to identify threshold values for improvement or deterioration, the reality is that it has been used predominantly to measure improvement. It turns out that most patients seeking care eventually improve! For this reason our discussion and examples are framed in the context of assessing improvement.

Typical DTM Study Design

DTM aims to identify a threshold value that accurately classifies patients as having improved or not. The typical study design has a group of patients with the condition and characteristics of interest being assessed at two points in time. The sample composition and interval between assessments are chosen such that some patients will undergo improvement and others will not. In addition to the outcome measure of interest, a reference standard is applied to distinguish patients who have truly improved from those who have not improved. Reference standards include retrospective global ratings of change,[13] prognostic ratings of change,[14] and concurrent ratings of change.[15] The final step taken by the researcher is to identify the change score on the outcome measure that best classifies patients as having improved or not.

How a Threshold Value Is Calculated from DTM Studies

The usual analysis involves building a 2 × 2 (read as "2 by 2") table similar to the one shown in Figure 6-2 for each change score obtained for the outcome measure under investigation.

The next step taken by a researcher is to calculate the sensitivity and specificity values for the change score associated with each 2 × 2 table. Applied in the context of diagnosing change, sensitivity represents those patients correctly labeled as improved by the outcome measure for a given change score divided by all patients identified by the reference standard as being truly improved ($a/(a + c)$). Specificity defines those patients correctly labeled as unimproved by the outcome measure for a given change score divided by all patients identified by the reference standard as being truly unimproved ($d/(b + d)$). Notice that sensitivity and specificity represent "vertical" calculations. Once sensitivity and specificity values have been calculated for all 2 × 2 tables, a receiver operating characteristic (ROC) curve is created. A ROC curve plots sensitivity on the *y*-axis against 1 minus specificity on the *x*-axis. The area under the curve (AUC) can be interpreted as a validity index. The greater the AUC, the more adept a measure is at distinguishing between patients who have improved from patients who have not improved. The AUC can vary from 0 to 1. An AUC of 0.50 indicates a measure does no better than chance at correctly labeling a patient's change

		Reference Standard True Improvement		
		Yes	No	
Outcome Measure Interpretation of Improvement	Yes	a	b	a + b
	No	c	d	c + d
		a + c	b + d	n = a + b + c + d

Prevalence or premeasure chance of improvement = the number of patients achieving an improvement (a + c) divided by all patients taking part in the study (n).

Sensitivity = the number of patients the measure correctly identifies as having achieved an improvement (a) divided by all patients who truly achieved an improvement (a + c).

Specificity = the number of patients the measure correctly identifies as not having achieved an improvement (d) divided by all patients who truly did not achieve an improvement (b + d).

Positive predictive value = the number of patients the measure correctly identifies as having achieved an improvement (a) divided by all patients identified by the measure as having achieved an improvement (a + b).

Negative predictive value = the number of patients the measure correctly identifies as not having achieved an improvement (d) divided by all patients identified by the measure as not having achieved an improvement (c + d).

Figure 6-2 Illustration of a 2 × 2 Table Used to Summarize the Results from a Diagnostic Test Study

status. Figure 6-3 provides results for a hypothetical outcome measure that has five change scores (i.e., −1, 0, 1, 2, 3). Figure 6-4 displays the ROC curve obtained by plotting sensitivity against 1 minus specificity. Also shown in this figure are the change score threshold values used to generate each 2 × 2 table.

When used to identify a threshold change value for clinical applications, researchers have uniformly equated the best threshold value with the change score that jointly maximizes sensitivity and specificity. It turns out that the change score associated with the data point on the ROC curve closest to the upper left corner of the graph represents the joint maximization of sensitivity and specificity. For example, in Figure 6-4 the change score of ≥2 yields the joint maximization of sensitivity and specificity with values of 91% and 89%, respectively.

		True Improvement			True Improvement			True Improvement			True Improvement			True Improvement	
		Yes	No		Yes	No		Yes	No		Yes	No		Yes	No
Measures	≥3	41	1	≥3	41	1	≥2	91	11	≥1	97	33	≥0	100	100
Change	2	50	10	<3	59	99	<2	9	89	<1	3	67	-1	0	0
Score	1	6	22												
	0	3	67												
	-1	0	0												
Total		100	100		100	100		100	100		100	100		100	100
Sensitivity					41%			91%			97%			100%	
Specificity						99%			89%			67%			0%

Figure 6-3 Illustration of the Effect of Different Change Scores on Sensitivity and Specificity

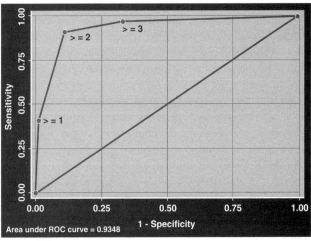

Figure 6-4 Receiver Operating Characteristic Curve

Translating DTM Results Into Clinically Useful Information: Sensitivity, Specificity, and Predictive Values

Recall from this chapter's introduction that a researcher knows a patient's true change status, whereas, a practicing physical therapist does not. When reporting results from DTM studies, researchers have often limited their reporting to threshold change estimates and sensitivity and specificity values. However, these values do not provide physical therapists with the chance of correctly labeling a patient as having improved or not.

The confidence in a clinical decision concerning a patient's change status is provided by the positive and negative predictive values. The positive predictive value represents those patients correctly labeled as improved by the outcome measure for a given change score divided by all patients identified by the outcome measure as having improved ($a/(a + b)$) (see Fig. 6-2). The negative predictive value denotes those patients correctly labeled as unimproved by the outcome measure for a given change score divided by all patients identified by the outcome measure as unimproved ($d/(c + d)$) (see Fig. 6-2).

An important nuance is that unlike sensitivity and specificity, predictive values are influenced by the prevalence or pre-measure chance of improvement. An increase in the pre-measure chance of improvement is accompanied by an increase in the positive predictive value and a decrease in the negative predictive value. As the pre-measure chance of improvement decreases, the positive predictive value decreases and the negative predictive value increases. In a diagnostic accuracy study, prevalence or the pre-measure chance of improvement defines the number of patients who truly achieved an improvement divided by all patients taking part in the study ($(a + c)/(a + b + c + d)$) (see Fig. 6-2). Stated another way, prevalence describes the chance a patient taking part in a study had of achieving an improvement prior to the application and interpretation of the outcome measure of interest. In clinical practice, the pre-measure chance of improvement can be thought of as the chance a physical therapist assigns to a patient of improving prior to administering the outcome measure and interpreting a patient's change score. To ascertain the positive and negative predictive values for a specific patient, a physical therapist must combine the sensitivity and specificity from a relevant study with the therapist's a priori assigned chance that a patient has improved.[16,17]

		Global Rating of Change True Improvement		
		Yes	No	
NDI Change Score	≥7.5	76	28	104
	<7.5	24	72	96
		100	100	200

Figure 6-5 Summary 2 × 2 Table for Predictive Value Calculation for a Pre-measure Chance of Improvement of 50%

A variation on the approach described above makes use of likelihood ratios. Likelihood ratios also combine information from sensitivity and specificity. The positive likelihood (LR+) is calculated as sensitivity divided by 1 minus specificity. The negative likelihood (LR–) is calculated as 1 minus sensitivity divided by specificity. These likelihood ratios are combined with the pre-measure chance of improvement to yield the post-measure chance of improvement given the threshold value has or has not been met. The post-measure chance of improvement given the threshold value has been met is identical to the positive predictive value. However, unlike the negative predictive value, the post-measure chance of improvement given the threshold value has not been met provides the chance that a patient has improved. As such it is equal to 1 minus the negative predictive value.

In Table 6-1 and Figure 6-5 we illustrate the calculation of predictive values using the results from the study by Young et al described below.[18] Other than grasping the interpretation of predictive values and post-measure chance of improvement, don't get too excited about the calculations. We have found a neat app for mobile devices that does a slick job of calculating both predictive values and post-measure chance of improvement. This app is called twoBytwo.*

---

* Ferguson, C. (2012). twoBytwo (Version1.1) [Computer Software]. Manchester, UK: Emmed Apps.

Table 6-1	Steps in Calculating Predictive Values for a Defined Pre-measure Chance of Improvement of 50%: Applying the Results from Young et al[18]

Step	Action	Example
1	Choose a convenient conceptual sample size (n).	In this example we chose an n of 200.
2	Fill in the $a + c$ by multiplying n by the pre-measure chance of achieving an improvement.	In this example we apply a 50% chance of improvement. 50% of 200 = 100. $a + c = 100$
3	Calculate $b + d$ by subtracting $a + c$ from n.	$b + d = 200 - 100 = 100$
4	Calculate a by multiplying $a + c$ by the sensitivity.	76% of 100 = 76. $a = 76$
5	Calculate c by subtracting a from $a + c$.	$c = 100 - 76 = 24$
6	Calculate d by multiplying $b + d$ by the specificity.	72% of 100 = 72. $d = 72$
7	Calculate b by subtracting d from $b + d$.	$b = 100 - 72 = 28$
8	Calculate the positive predictive value as $[100\% \times a/(a + b)]$.	$[100\% \times a/(a + b)] = 100\% \times 76/104 = 73\%$
9	Calculate the negative predictive value as $[100\% \times d/(c + d)]$.	$[100\% \times d/(c + d)] = 100\% \times 72/96 = 75\%$

The results from these calculations are shown in Figure 6-5. Notice that the predictive values have changed from those reported in Figure 6-6 for a study prevalence of 72%.

		Global Rating of Change True Improvement		
		Yes	No	
NDI Change Score	≥7.5	50	7	57
	<7.5	16	18	34
		66	25	91

Study Specific Results

Prevalence =   =   72%
Sensitivity =   =   76%
Specificity =   =   72%
Positive predictive value =   88%
Negative predictive value =   53%

Post-measure chance of improvement given threshold values has been met ≥ 7.5 = 88%. Post-measure chance of improvement given threshold values has not been met ≥7.5 = 47%.

Results adjusted to a premeasure chance of improvement of 50% (see chapter appendix for calculation).

Positive predictive value =   73%
Negative predictive value =   75%

Post-measure chance of improvement given threshold values has been met ≥ 7.5 = 73%. Post-measure chance of improvement given threshold values has not been met ≥7.5 = 25%.

Figure 6-6 Approximate Results from Young et al[18]

A Clinical Example | **Based on a Study by Young et al: Predictive Value Method[18]**

Young et al sought to identify a threshold improvement value for the Neck Disability Index (NDI).[18] The NDI is a 10-item, region-specific, self-report questionnaire that combines impairments and activities. Each item is scored 0 to 5, with higher scores representing greater amounts of pain-related activities. Total scores can vary from 0 to 50. Young et al applied the NDI to 91 patients with neck pain at their initial assessment and following 3 weeks of treatment. Also administered at the 3-week follow-up visit was a global rating of change (GRC) scale that classified patients as improved, unchanged, or worsened. Young et al applied a ROC curve analysis that defined the threshold value for improvement as the change score that jointly maximized sensitivity and specificity. Sixty-six patients were labeled by the GRC as truly improved, 25 as truly unchanged, and zero as worsened. The threshold value for improvement was 7.5 NDI improvement points and the AUC was 0.79. Young et al did not identify the exact values for sensitivity and specificity in the publication; however, it is possible to approximate them from a figure provided in their manuscript. Referring to Figure 2 of their publication, we estimated the sensitivity and specificity to be 0.76 and 0.72, respectively. Applying these values we constructed the 2 × 2 table shown in Figure 6-6 and calculated the study-specific (i.e., based on the study's prevalence of improvement of 72.5% [66/91]) positive and negative predictive values to be 88% and 53%, respectively.

How the Physical Therapist Applied the Information

A physical therapist applied the NDI to Mr. Smith, a patient with neck pain and restricted range of motion. Mr. Smith's initial NDI score was 22/50 and his reassessment value was 13/50. The physical therapist believed that Mr. Smith had a 50% chance of improving prior to administering the NDI at his reassessment. Combining a pre-measure chance of improvement of 50% with sensitivity and specificity values of 76% and 72%, respectively, yielded a positive predictive value of 73% and a negative predictive value of 75% (see Table 6-1 for calculation). The physical therapist interpreted Mr. Smith's 9-point change as a true improvement. Applying the NDI coupled with the results from Young et al has increased the physical therapist's confidence that Mr. Smith has improved from 50% to 73%.

▶ Unchanged Group Method of Estimating a Threshold Value for Change

The unchanged group approach is a widely used method for estimating a threshold value for true change commonly referred to as the minimal detectable change (MDC). MDC is a variation on the Reliability Change Index proposed by Jacobson and colleagues,[19,20] and we briefly describe the difference between these quantities later in this chapter. MDC is based on unchanged patients only and its goal is to quantify the variability in responses of truly unchanged patients when an outcome measure is administered on two occasions. MDC is based on the notion that if there is a small chance that a patient's change score is consistent with the typical difference scores between test and retest of truly unchanged patients, then it's likely that a patient has changed.

Typical Unchanged Group Study Design

The unchanged group estimation method applies a test-retest reliability study design identical to that discussed in Chapter 4. Patients with the condition and characteristics of interest are assessed on two occasions and the difference between responses is used to estimate MDC. Two essential assumptions associated with this design are (1) patients' true values for the outcome of interest have not changed and (2) the distribution of patients' difference scores between test and retest is consistent with a normal distribution. These are the same requirements mentioned in Chapter 4 when estimating the error for a measured score value.

How a Threshold Value Is Calculated from Unchanged Group Studies

A researcher calculates MDC by building a distribution of difference scores between test and retest for unchanged patients. Provided the distribution of difference scores is consistent with a normal distribution, the standard deviation of the difference values (SD_{diff}) is then calculated. SD_{diff} represents the variability between test and retest values averaged across all patients taking part in the study. Assuming a normal distribution, 68% of patients would display random fluctuations between test and retest of ± 1 SD_{diff}. When reporting MDC it is common to specify a confidence level, which is frequently conveyed using a subscript. For example, MDC_{68} signifies a 68% confidence level. Often, one desires a greater confidence level and this is accomplished by multiplying SD_{diff} by the z-value* associated with the confidence level of interest. For instance, if we were interested in a 90% confidence level, SD_{diff} would be multiplied by 1.65, where 1.65 is the z-value associated with a two-tailed 90% confidence level. Although the choice of confidence level is arbitrary, 90% and 95% levels are typically reported by researchers. A relationship worth remembering is that SD_{diff} is equal to the standard error of measurement (SEM) times $\sqrt{2}$. Thus, a researcher could also calculate MDC at a particular confidence level as follows: SEM $\times \sqrt{2} \times$ z-value associated with the confidence level of interest. The $\sqrt{2}$ term acknowledges that error is associated with the previous and current assessments' values.

Translating MDC into Clinically Useful Information

Although researchers frequently report MDC, its direct application to clinical decision-making is extremely limited. To explain this statement we return to Figure 6-1 and the challenge faced by a physical therapist when making a decision concerning a patient's change status. MDC is based on unchanged patients. These patients would be represented in the right hand, or unimproved, column of Figure 6-1. Because information concerning truly improved patients is unavailable, we cannot determine the chance that a patient with a given change score has improved or not. Applying MDC, a patient's change score can be interpreted only from the perspective that a patient is truly unchanged. For example, the interpretation of MDC_{90} is that 90% of truly unchanged patients will display random fluctuations equal to or less than this value. MDC does not provide the chance that a patient with a given change score has changed, nor does it stipulate the chance that a patient with a given change score has not changed.

---

* The z-value is a standard score which is referenced to the standard normal or Z distribution.

A Clinical Example Unchanged Group Methodology Based on a Study by Huang et al[21]

To emphasize the connection between MDC and test-retest reliability studies, we return to the study by Huang et al mentioned in Chapter 4.[21] One purpose of their study was to estimate MDC_{95} for the Timed-Up-and-Go (TUG) test for patients with Parkinson disease attending a specialty clinic for movement disorders at a university hospital. Seventy-two patients fulfilling the eligibility criteria were assessed on two occasions approximately 2 weeks apart. These patients' true TUG times were believed to be unchanged over this interval. The mean (SD) difference between test and retest was 0 (2.0) seconds. MDC_{95} can be calculated as 2.0 seconds × 1.96, where 1.96 is the z-value for a 95% confidence level. Thus, MDC_{95} is 3.9 seconds.

How the Physical Therapist Applied the Information

Mr. Park is a patient being treated by a physical therapist in a movement disorder clinic. Mr. Park's characteristics are similar to those of the patients who took part in the study by Huang et al.[21] Two months ago Mr. Park's TUG time was 12.2 seconds. Today, his TUG time is 13.8 seconds. Mr. Park's physical therapist wonders whether this difference is likely to represent a true worsening in performance. Applying the results from the study of Huang et al, the physical therapist interprets the difference in Mr. Park's TUG times as being consistent with the variability in TUG times seen in truly unchanged patients and does not interpret the apparent difference as a true worsening in performance. The physical therapist, however, realizes that the study by Huang et al does not provide information that can be translated into the chance that the decision of no change is the correct decision.

◗ Reliability Change Index and Minimal Detectable Change

The Reliability Change Index (RCI) was conceived to determine whether the observed magnitude of change for a patient is statistically reliable. Whereas MDC provides a threshold value for change based on an arbitrary confidence level, RCI expresses the observed change as a probability. Referring to the previous example, we saw that the difference in Mr. Park's TUG times of 1.6 seconds did not meet the MDC_{95} value of 3.9 seconds. However, the MDC does not provide the exact chance that a truly unchanged patient will display a difference equal to or greater than the measured difference (e.g., 1.6 seconds for Mr. Park). The RCI overcomes this limitation by calculating this probability as follows:

$$RCI = \frac{current\ value - previous\ value}{SD_{diff}}$$

where the value for RCI represents a z-value that is referred to in the standard normal distribution tables found in statistical textbooks. For Mr. Park, the RCI is

$$RCI = \frac{13.8 - 12.2}{2}$$
$$RCI = 0.80$$
$$Z = 0.80$$

Comparing a z-value of 0.80 to the standard normal distribution, we find the probability of obtaining a difference of ± 1.6 seconds or more in truly unchanged patients is 0.42. Stated another way, 42% of truly unchanged patients will display differences between two measurements of ± 1.6 seconds or more.

MDC and RCI have their own strengths and limitations. For MDC, no calculation is required; however, the choice of confidence level is arbitrary. For RCI, the exact confidence level is obtained; however, a calculation and ready access to the standard normal probability table are required. Like MDC, RCI does not provide the chance that a patient with a given change score has improved.

▶ Percentile Improvement Method of Estimating a Threshold Value for Change

The percentile improvement method (PIM) is based solely on the change values of patients who, according to a reference standard, have truly improved.[1] The PIM is founded on the premise that if there is a reasonably good chance a patient's improvement score is consistent with the improvement scores of truly improved patients, then a patient is considered to have improved. Like DTM, the PIM can be used to identify threshold values for true improvement and clinically important improvement, depending on the reference standard for change. Of the three methods discussed in this chapter, PIM appears least often in the literature.

Typical PIM Study Design

A cohort of patients with the condition and characteristics of interest is assessed at two points in time. The interval between assessments is selected such that many patients should truly improve. From the original cohort, a subsample of improved patients is identified by the reference standard.

How a Threshold Value Is Calculated from PIM Studies

The analysis is restricted to patients who, according to the reference standard, have improved. The first step taken by the researcher is to create a change score for each patient by calculating the difference between initial and follow-up measurements. Next, the change scores are ordered from lowest to highest to create a distribution of change scores. Prior to undertaking the analysis, the researcher declares a percentile rank that will be used to reference the threshold for improvement. Like the selection of the confidence level for MDC, the choice of percentile is arbitrary. For example, in a landmark publication Goldsmith and colleagues applied the 25th percentile.[1] Patients with outcome measure change scores equal to or greater than that of the 25th percentile are considered to have truly improved. Because the threshold value is based on a percentile rank, the distribution of change scores need not be consistent with a normal distribution.

Translating PIM Results into Clinically Useful Information

Like MDC, the direct application of PIM to clinical decision-making is limited. The reason for this is that PIM considers improved patients only. Once again referring to Figure 6-1, we see that PIM's estimated threshold value for improvement is ascertained by applying information in the improved column only. Because PIM's reference frame is patients known to have truly improved, it is incapable of providing the chance that a patient with a given change score has improved or worsened.

A Clinical Example | **PIM Based on a Study by Goldsmith et al[1]**

In a novel study, Goldsmith et al sought to identify threshold values for clinically important improvement for a number of outcome measures relevant to patients with rheumatoid arthritis (RA).[1] Rather than using real patients, Goldsmith et al developed 64 patient profiles that provided information on swollen joint count (scored 0 to 66), tender joint count (scored 0 to 68), pain (0–10), patient global assessment (0–10), physician global assessment (scored 0–10), and disability (scored 0–10). Each profile consisted of initial and follow-up values separated by 6 to 12 months, during which time patients were taking a drug with a toxicity level similar to low-dose oral methotrexate. The patient profiles were constructed in such a way as to represent responses obtained from real patients. The profiles were presented to teams of raters and a consensus process was used to ascertain whether each profile represented an important improvement. Of the 64 patient profiles, 35 were deemed to have undergone an important improvement. Prior to examining the data, the researchers defined the 25th percentile as the threshold percentile for an important improvement. Applying this standard, an important improvement for a patient measured on the 0- to 10-point disability scale was a change of 3.6 points.

How the Physical Therapist Applied the Information

Mr. Smith is a patient with RA who has clinical characteristics similar to profile patients reported in Goldsmith et al's study. Mr. Smith's initial disability rating was 8/10 (higher values represent more disability). Following 4 weeks of physiotherapy, his disability rating is 4/10. Mr. Smith's physical therapist interprets the 4-point change in disability as an important improvement. This interpretation is based on the understanding that 75% patients who truly improve an important amount will display a change in disability of 3.6 points or more. The physical therapist understands that the study by Goldsmith et al does not provide the chance that a patient reporting an improvement of 4 or more points has truly improved an important amount.

▶ Putting It All Together: A Direct Comparison of the Three Threshold Value Estimation Methods

In this section we use a common dataset to illustrate the information provided by the three estimation methods described previously. We apply a vignette that incorporates a hypothetical measure that we have named the New Upper Extremity Functional Scale (NUEFS). The vignette consists of a hypothetical study that estimates threshold NUEFS improvement values and a clinical scenario that applies the information provided by the study.

■ Vignette: Hypothetical Study Summary

Purpose: The purpose of this study was to estimate improvement threshold values using DTM, MDC_{90}, and PIM for the NUEFS when applied to patients with lateral epicondylitis at the elbow.

Methods: The study sample consisted of 160 patients with a clinical diagnosis of lateral epicondylitis at the elbow. The NUEFS was applied to patients at their initial assessment and following 3 weeks of physical therapy treatment that consisted of exercise and pulsed ultrasound. The NUEFS is scored on a 0- to 25-point scale, with higher values representing higher levels of functional status. Also applied at the follow-up visit was a retrospective global rating of change that served as the reference standard. The researcher calculated threshold values for true improvement using DTM, PIM, and MDC_{90}. For DTM, the threshold value for true improvement was defined as the change score that jointly maximized sensitivity and specificity. For PIM, the 25th percentile was selected to define the threshold value for improvement. And for MDC_{90}, the threshold value for improvement was calculated by multiplying the standard deviation of the difference score by 1.65, the z-value associated with a 90% confidence level.

Results: Of the 160 patients, the reference standard identified 100 as truly improved and 60 as truly unchanged. This represents a study prevalence or pre-measure chance of improvement of 62.5%. The mean (SD) NUEFS change score for the improved group was 4.6 (2.8) points compared to 0 (2.5) for the unchanged group. Table 6-2 reports the sensitivity and specificity values for the various NUEFS change scores obtained from the study sample. Sensitivity and specificity were jointly maximized with values of 78.0% and 83.3%, respectively, for a NUEFS threshold improvement score of ≥3 (Fig. 6-7). Applying the PIM, the 25th percentile corresponded to an improvement of 3 NUEFS points. MDC_{90} was calculated to be 4.6 points. Figure 6-8 shows the distribution of NUEFS change scores for truly improved and unimproved patients along with the number of patients correctly classified using a threshold value of ≥3 (solid line extending across both panels indicates cut-point). Also presented in this figure are the PIM (left panel) and MDC_{90} (right panel) threshold values. In this example the three methods produced similar threshold values for change; however, this will not always be the case.

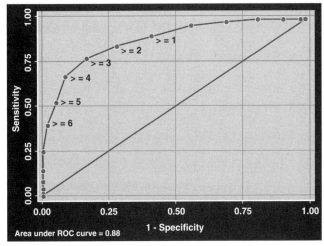

Figure 6-7 ROC Curve for NUEFS Change Scores

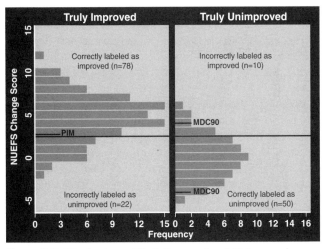

Figure 6-8 Distributions of Truly Improved and Unimproved Patients with PIM and MDC$_{90}$ Values Superimposed on the Distributions

Clinical Application

Mrs. Crowe is a patient with lateral epicondylitis at the elbow. Her initial NUEFS value was 12. Following 2 weeks of treatment with pulsed ultrasound and exercise, Mrs. Crowe was reassessed and obtained a score of 17. The physical therapist chose a 2-week reassessment interval based on his experience that approximately 50% of patients with characteristics similar to Mrs. Crowe undergo a true improvement over this interval. The physical therapist wondered whether the measured 5-point improvement was likely to represent a true improvement. This question can be answered two ways. First, the physical therapist realized that only DTM is capable of providing the chance that a patient with a specified change score has improved or not. Accordingly, the physical therapist focused on the results specific to DTM. Seeing that Mrs. Crowe's change score exceeded the DTM threshold value of 3, the therapist interpreted Mrs. Crowe as having truly improved. To support this impression, the therapist calculated the positive predictive value to be 82% by combining Mrs. Crowe's assigned pre-measure chance of improvement (i.e., 50%) with sensitivity and specificity values of 78.0% and 83.3%, respectively. However, this positive predictive value applies to patients with NUEFS improvement scores of 3 or more. Given Mrs. Crowe 5-point improvement, the therapist went on to recalculate the positive predictive value for patients improving 5 or more points. This was done by combining the patient-specific pre-measure chance of improvement—once again, 50%—with the sensitivity and specificity values for an improvement of ≥5 points. Referring to Table 6-2, we see the sensitivity and specificity values for an improvement of ≥5 points are 53% and 95%, respectively. Combining this information yields a positive predictive value of 91%, and the physical therapist concluded with a high level of confidence that Mrs. Crowe had truly improved.

Table 6-2 Number of Truly Improved and Unimproved Patients and Sensitivity and Specificity Values for NUEFS Change Scores

NUEFS Change Score	Sensitivity (%)	Specificity (%)	Truly Improved	Truly Unimproved
≥−5	100.0	0	0	0
≥−4	100.0	1.7	0	1
≥−3	100.0	8.3	0	4
≥−2	100.0	18.3	1	6
≥−1	99.0	30.0	2	7
≥0	97.0	43.3	6	8
≥1	91.0	58.3	6	9
≥2	85.0	71.7	7	8
≥3	**78.0**	**83.3**	10	7
≥4	68.0	91.7	15	5
≥5	53.0	95.0	13	2
≥6	40.0	98.3	15	2
≥7	25.0	100.0	11	1
≥8	14.0	100.0	6	0
≥9	8.0	100.0	4	0
≥10	4.0	100.0	3	0
≥12	1.0	100.0	1	0

▶ Considerations When Assessing Clinically Important Change

When discussing change with a patient, the literature distinguishes between true change and clinically important change, the idea being that it is possible for a patient to undergo a true change without it being clinically important. For example, it's possible for a patient to undergo a true improvement in knee flexion range of motion without the increased range translating into improvements in activities such as climbing stairs or cycling. Jaeschke and colleagues defined the minimal clinically important difference (MCID) as "the smallest difference in score in the domain of interest which patients perceive as beneficial and which would mandate, in the absence of troublesome side effects and excessive cost, a change in the patient's management."[13] In this section we introduce several important points to consider when contemplating clinically important change.

There's a Difference Between a Within-Patient Change and Between-Group Difference

This text's focus is on clinical decision-making applied to individual patients. In this chapter, we have reviewed several methods commonly used to estimate an important within-patient change. However, the interpretation of an important within-patient change is drastically different from that of an important between-group difference. An important within-patient change is of interest to clinicians treating individual patients. An important between-group difference is of interest to researchers conducting and interpreting the results of clinical trials. At times this distinction has gone unnoticed.

There is now good evidence to suggest that an important within-patient change is substantially greater than an important between-group difference.[1,2] Goldsmith and colleagues were perhaps the first to show this.[1] These investigators estimated an important within-patient change to be 36% of a patient's baseline value, compared to 18% for an important between-group difference. Similarly, Roland and Fairbank noted that a within-patient change of 5 points on the Roland-Morris questionnaire is important and a between-group difference of 2 points is important.[2] Applying the magnitude of an important between-group difference to individual patients will result in labeling an increased number of patients as having changed when it fact they have not.

Minimal Clinically Important Improvement in the Context of Specific Interventions

To this point, we have focused on an important change as a property of an outcome measure without considering the context in which the measure is applied. In clinical practice, outcome measures are typically used to monitor the progress of patients over the course of treatment. Often, a number of potential interventions are available for the same patient problem. However, these competing interventions may not present the same cost, level of convenience, and risk of an adverse event. Presumably, increases in cost, inconvenience, or risk of an adverse event would mandate larger important change values.[5] At the time of writing this text we could not find a study in the physical therapy literature that identified estimates of important change specific to interventions that carried different costs, risks, or levels of inconvenience. However, Goldsmith et al, in the example provided in the PIM section, equated the toxicity level of the drug under consideration to be similar to low-dose oral methotrexate.[1] This is one of the few articles in the medical literature that has considered risks and harm when estimating an important within-patient change or between-group difference.

Minimal Clinically Important Improvement Is Baseline Score Dependent

Although the amount of change necessary to be deemed clinically important is usually reported as a single value, we now know that its magnitude is related to the value of a patient's previous assessment.[1,6–8] To be considered clinically important it turns out that a greater change is required in patients who are worse off.[6–9] There are three likely explanations for this phenomenon. Jacobson proposed that for a change to be considered clinically important a patient's health state must move from a dysfunctional to a functional state.[20] Thus, patients who present with lower functioning levels must undergo a greater change to reach a functional state than patients who initially display higher functioning levels. The second reason is a consequence of measuring the outcome of interest on a bounded scale. By this we mean a scale that has defined upper and lower limits, such as the 0- to 10-point numeric pain rating scale. For example, a patient who initially reports a pain score of 2/10 can improve only 2 points, whereas a patient who presents with a score of 8/10 has the potential to improve 8 points.

The third reason is related to the measurement concept known as regression towards the mean.[22] The explanation for this concept is tied to the notion of random measurement error that was introduced in Chapter 4. One reason many patients present with extremely high scores is that the measurement error is pulling their scores towards the extreme of the scale range. Given that measurement error is random, many patients who initially presented with extremely high scores will tend to report lower scores on reassessment even though their true scores have not changed. Conversely, patients who initially reported extremely low scores will tend to report higher scores on reassessment even though their true status has not changed. If, for example, an important change was 5 points for patients with previous assessment values in the midrange of a scale, a patient with a large limitation in the outcome of interest would have to improve 5 points plus the error associated with regression towards the mean. For example, if the error associated with regression towards the mean was an apparent increase in a patient's value of 2 points, we would expect an important change for this patient to be 5 + 2, or 7 points. A similar explanation can be offered for patients who had previous assessment values that display small limitations in the outcome of interest; however, in this case the effect of regression towards the mean would be subtracted from the change value for the midrange important improvement value (e.g., 5 − 2, or 3 points). It is likely that in many instances all three of these explanations are present to some extent.

If clinically important change is dependent on the previous assessment's value, why do researchers report a single value? There are several possible explanations. The idea of an important difference originated in the context of clinical trials where the goal was to compare the effectiveness of competing interventions. Typically, the measure of relative effect was a single value, the average between-group difference for the outcome of interest. With this history in mind, it is likely that early on it did not occur to investigators that a clinically important within-patient improvement would be score dependent. This is particularly true for studies conducted over a decade ago. Another possible explanation is that a single value for clinically important improvement works reasonably well for many patients seen in clinical practice provided their scores are not near the extremes of the scale range.

Given that the threshold value for an important change varies depending on a patient's previous value, how can physical therapists incorporate this added complexity into their decision-making process? The simplest approach is to apply the recommended single value, and this would seem reasonable in instances where patients' scores lie between the 25th and 75th percentile points of the scale range. A second strategy is to apply a "rule-of-thumb" guideline that defines the magnitude of an important change as a percentage of the maximum possible improvement score. By maximum possible improvement score we mean the difference between a patient's previous assessment value and the maximum possible positive health state score.

To clarify this point, consider a patient who has a pain score of 3/10, where 0 is no pain, and a function score of 3/10, where 10 is full function. If we consider a 35% change to be clinically important, the pain score would have to decrease by 1.05 points (i.e., 3×0.35, where 3 is the difference between 3 and 0), whereas the function score would have to increase by 2.45 points (i.e., 7×0.35, where 7 is the difference between 3 and 10). Although no single rule-of-thumb percentage has achieved universal acceptance, suggested values are typically between 30% and 36%.[1,8,10] A third and perhaps more desirable approach is to seek out studies that have provided measure- and context-specific estimates of an important change across the scale range for the measure of interest.[6,7] One suggested guideline has been to generate clinically important change estimates for tertiles of the baseline score.[23]

Chapter Summary

- In clinical practice a physical therapist must decide whether a change score is likely to represent a truly changed or unchanged patient.

- Of the three threshold value estimation methods, only DTM answers the question "What is the chance that a patient with a given change score has truly improved or not improved?"

- DTM provides a threshold change score that maximizes the correct classification of patients as having improved or not.

- MDC provides an estimate of true change by quantifying the variability in truly unchanged patients.

- MDC does *not* answer the question "What is the chance that a patient with a given change score has truly improved or not improved?"

- Because many DTM studies have focused on improvement only, in many instances MDC currently provides the best guide for determining whether a patient has worsened.

- PIM provides an estimate of improvement based on truly changed patients only.

- PIM defines a threshold change score based on a declared percentile value.

- PIM and DTM can be applied to estimate true improvement and important improvement.

- The minimal clinically important improvement (MCII) is greater for individual patient decisions compared to between-intervention group decisions.

- For a given measure and intervention combination, MCII is likely to increase as the costs and risks associated with the intervention increase.

- MCII is score dependent.

■ Reference List

1. Goldsmith CH, Boers M, Bombardier C, Tugwell P. Criteria for clinically important changes in outcomes: Development, scoring and evaluation of rheumatoid arthritis patient and trial profiles. OMERACT Committee. *J Rheumatol* 1993;20:561–5.

2. Roland M, Fairbank J. The Roland-Morris Disability Questionnaire and the Oswestry Disability Questionnaire. *Spine* 2000;25:3115–24.

3. Barrett B, Brown R, Mundt M, Dye L, Alt J, Safdar N, et al. Using benefit harm tradeoffs to estimate sufficiently important difference: The case of the common cold. *Med Decis Making* 2005;25:47–55.

4. Barrett B, Brown D, Mundt M, Brown R. Sufficiently important difference: Expanding the framework of clinical significance. *Med Decis Making* 2005;25:250–61.

5. Ferreira ML, Herbert RD. What does "clinically important" really mean? *Aust J Physiother* 2008;54:229–30.

6. Stratford PW, Binkley JM, Riddle DL, Guyatt GH. Sensitivity to change of the Roland-Morris Back Pain Questionnaire: Part 1. *Phys Ther* 1998; 78:1186–96.

7. Riddle DL, Stratford PW, Binkley JM. Sensitivity to change of the Roland-Morris Back Pain Questionnaire: Part 2. *Phys Ther* 1998;78: 1197–207.

8. Ostelo RW, Deyo RA, Stratford P, Waddell G, Croft P, Von Korff M, et al. Interpreting change scores for pain and functional status in low back pain: Towards international consensus regarding minimal important change. *Spine* 2008;33:90–4.

9. Wang YC, Hart DL, Stratford PW, Mioduski JE. Baseline dependency of minimal clinically important improvement. *Phys Ther* 2011;95: 675–88.

10. Farrar JT, Young JP, Jr., LaMoreaux L, Werth JL, Poole RM. Clinical importance of changes in chronic pain intensity measured on an 11-point numerical pain rating scale. *Pain* 2001;94:149–58.

11. Peterson WW, Birdshall TG, Fox WC. The theory of signal detectability. IRE Transactions: Professional Group on Information Theory, 1954;4: 171–212.

12. Deyo RA, Centor RM. Assessing the responsiveness of functional scales to clinical change: An analogy to diagnostic test performance. *J Chronic Dis* 1986;39:897–906.

13. Jaeschke R, Singer J, Guyatt GH. Measurement of health status. Ascertaining the minimal clinically important difference. *Control Clin Trials* 1989;10:407–15.

14. Westaway MD, Stratford PW, Binkley JM. The patient-specific functional scale: Validation of its use in persons with neck dysfunction. *J Orthop Sports Phys Ther* 1998;27:331–8.

15. Fletcher KE, French CT, Irwin RS, Corapi KM, Norman GR. A prospective global measure, the Punum Ladder, provides more valid assessments of quality of life than a retrospective transition measure. *J Clin Epidemiol* 2010;63:1123–31.

16. Stratford PW, Riddle DL, Binkley JM. Assessing for changes in a patient's status: A review of current methods and a proposal for a new method of estimating true change. *Physiother Can* 2001;53:175–81.

17. Stratford PW. Diagnosing patient change: Impact of reassessment interval. *Physiother Can* 2000;52:225–8.

18. Young BA, Walker MJ, Strunce JB, Boyles RE, Whitman JM, Childs JD. Responsiveness of the Neck Disability Index in patients with mechanical neck disorders. *Spine J* 2009;9:802–8.

19. Jacobson NS, Follette WC, Revenstorf D, Baucom DH, Hahlweg K, Margolin G. Variability in outcome and clinical significance of behavioral marital therapy: A reanalysis of outcome data. *J Consult Clin Psychol* 1984;52:497–504.

20. Jacobson NS, Truax P. Clinical significance: A statistical approach to defining meaningful change in psychotherapy research. *J Consult Clin Psychol* 1991;59:12–9.

21. Huang SL, Hsieh CL, Wu RM, Tai CH, Lin CH, Lu WS. Minimal detectable change of the timed up & go test and the dynamic gait index in people with Parkinson disease. *Phys Ther* 2011;91:114–21.

22. Stratford PW, Spadoni GF. Assessing improvement in patients who report small limitations in functional status on condition-specific measures. *Physiother Can* 2005;57:234–41.

23. Tubach F, Ravaud P, Baron G, Falissard B, Logeart I, Bellamy N, et al. Evaluation of clinically relevant changes in patient reported outcomes in knee and hip osteoarthritis: The minimal clinically important improvement. *Ann Rheum Dis* 2005;64:29–33.

Chapter 7

How Can I Establish a Target Goal Value for My Patient?

■ *Therapists are routinely faced with the challenge of making prognostic judgments for their patients. For example, patients often ask questions like "Will my back pain go away completely?" or "Will I be able to walk without this limp?" These types of questions are classic prognostic questions and are some of the most difficult to answer in patient care. In our view, they are difficult to answer for two main reasons: (1) the volume of literature on prognosis is less than that for other types of clinical decisions, particularly for certain disorders, and (2) these types of questions can be very broad in nature, which make it difficult to provide a clear and concise answer.*

What's Ahead

In the previous chapter we introduced three methods frequently used to identify a true or important change threshold or goal value. In this chapter we describe methods often used to establish target goal values. We use the term *target goal value* to denote the long-term or discharge value for the outcome of interest. An example of a target goal is as follows: To increase the patient's 20-m walk pace to 1.2 m/sec or more in 6 weeks. In this example the target goal value is 1.2 m/sec.

A Note on Terminology

For some patients seen by physical therapists a full recovery is expected. For other patients the expected recovery will be less than what one might anticipate for a person of similar age and gender in the population. In this chapter we apply the term *satis-factory outcome* to describe the expected optimal recovery given each patient's unique circumstance. For some patients this implies a complete recovery; for other patients it represents a state that is a less than complete recovery.

The Concept Behind This Question

A universal goal of physical therapy interventions is to optimize the functional status of patients. Central to this goal is the recognition that optimal function will be patient specific. This means that a target goal value will also be patient specific. Establishing well-conceived target goals draws heavily on the three pillars of evidence-based practice: patient's values, clinical experience, and best evidence.[1] The patient provides the physical therapist with expectations. The physical therapist considers these expectations within the unique context of each patient and seeks out the best prognostic evidence suggesting a target goal value.

▶ Methods Used to Establish Target Goal Values

The Within-Patient Comparison Approach

The reasoning behind the comparison approach is that in an otherwise healthy person the contralateral limb provides a patient-specific expectation for the target goal value. This approach is often used to establish target values for impairments such as restricted range of motion and reduced muscle strength. A variation of the approach is also popular when forming a target goal concerning the mobility of a compromised spinal motion segment. Here the mobility of the presumed normal motion segments above and below the motion segment of interest are used to guide the target goal value.

The within-patient comparison approach has strong face validity, but there is little research that actually validates it. For example, Petersen et al noted that the 10% grip strength rule—the dominant hand possesses 10% greater grip strength than the nondominant hand—applied to right-hand-dominant but not left-hand-dominant persons.[2] Also, Shultz and Nguyen found that side-to-side differences for a variety of lower extremity bony alignment characteristics exceeded measurement error in up to 32% of the subjects tested.[3] These data suggest that for some measurements, considerable variability in left-to-right differences exists in asymptomatic persons and it is best not to assume symmetry when making judgments about the meaningfulness of a side-to-side difference. Because this method of obtaining a goal value is self-evident, we will not elaborate further.

Normal or Customary Values: What Is It?

Normal or customary values typically provide information from population-based or large-sample studies. These normative or customary values are most useful when a patient's outcome is expected to be consistent with that of the typical person in the population.

Study Design

A representative sample of persons is identified and the outcome of interest is assessed at a single point in time.

How Customary Values Are Calculated

The usual analysis provides a measure of central tendency (i.e., mean or median) and variation (i.e., standard deviation or quartiles). Also, 95% confidence intervals for the estimated mean are typically reported. The results are usually stratified by potential predictor variables such as age or gender, and the stratum-specific central tendency value serves at the target goal value. A crucial assumption is that a representative and sufficiently large number of patients is sampled in order that a precise and accurate target value is obtained.

Interpretation

Persons with outcome measure values in close proximity (e.g., ±1 standard deviation) to the central tendency value or patients with values exceeding the central tendency value are viewed as having met their target goal.

The Bottom Line

A limitation of this method is that from a practical perspective it can take into consideration only a few classifying characteristics (e.g., age and gender). Accordingly, the identified target value may not be sufficiently specific for some patients. A variation on using the central tendency value is to apply a percentile approach, which we discuss in a subsequent portion of this chapter.

A Clinical Example | **What the Researcher Did**

To establish normative data for the Medical Outcomes Study 36-item Short Form (SF-36) generic health status measure,[4] Hopman et al conducted a prospective cohort study of 9,423 randomly selected Canadian men and women aged 25 years or more dwelling in the community.[5] The SF-36 assesses eight health concepts, consisting of physical functioning, role physical, bodily pain, general health perceptions, vitality, social functioning, role emotional, and mental health. Each health concept is scored on a 0- to 100-point scale, with higher scores representing more positive health states. Although Hopman et al reported age and gender standardized values for all eight health concepts, for the purpose of this example we report the physical functioning summary information for persons aged 55 to 64 years. This age-specific sample consisted of 2,282 persons. The mean (SD) physical functioning score was 82.3 (19.3) and the 95% confidence interval for the mean was 81.5 to 83.0.

How the Physical Therapist Applied the Information

Mrs. Jones is a 60 year old who is referred to physical therapy for reconditioning following 6 weeks of hospitalization with multiorgan failure of unknown origin. Organ functioning has been fully restored and a full recovery is expected. Because the extended hospitalization impacted many facets of Mrs. Jones's life, her physical therapist selected the SF-36 as one outcome measure. Although the physical therapist was interested in all of Mrs. Jones's SF-36 domain scores, for this example we focus on the physical functioning domain only. Acknowledging that Mrs. Jones was an active tennis player and hiker, the physical therapist set the target SF-36 physical functioning value at 83 points. Using similar reasoning, the physical therapist set goal values for each of the other seven SF-36 domains.

Reference Equations with Multiple Predictor Variables: What Is It?

Reference equations are derived from multiple regression models that consist of the outcome measure (dependent variable) and a number of independent variables used to predict the outcome measure's value.

Study Design

Similar to the previous design, a representative sample of persons is identified and the outcome of interest and potential predictor variables are assessed at the same point in time.

How Reference Equations Are Constructed

The association between the outcome or dependent variable and the potential predictor variables is modeled using multiple linear regression.[6] The general form of a multiple linear regression model is as follows:

$$\text{outcome measure score} = \beta_0 + \beta_1 \text{ (predictor1 score)} + \beta_2 \text{ (predictor2 score)} + \lambda$$

where β values are the regression coefficients.

There are two important conditions for a model to be valid. First, it is essential that a representative and sufficiently large number of patients be sampled in order to identify the predictor variables and their respective regression (β) coefficients. A second requirement is that the statistical assumptions associated with the specified model hold true. These assumptions vary depending on the model and a discussion of them is beyond the scope of this text.

Interpretation

The model provides an expected outcome target value for a given set of predictor variable values.

The Bottom Line

Reference equations share the advantages of normative value tables with one added benefit. Provided a sufficiently large and representative sample is used to build the model, reference equations can handle a greater number of predictor variables than is practical with the normal-value method described previously.

A Clinical Example **What the Researcher Did**

This example is based on a study by Enright and Sherrill.[7] These investigators modeled reference equations for 6MWD based on age (years), height (cm), and weight (kg). Their study sample consisted of 117 healthy men and 173 healthy women aged 40 to 80 years. The equations for men and women are as follows:

Men

6MWD = (7.57 × height cm) − (5.02 × age years) −
$$(1.76 \times \text{weight kg}) - 309 \text{ m}$$

Women

6MWD = 667 m + (2.11 × height cm) −
$$(5.78 \times \text{age years}) - (2.29 \times \text{weight kg})$$

How the Physical Therapist Applied the Information

Mr. Davis, an active 55 year old, experienced a mild stroke 8 weeks ago. Currently, he is receiving physical therapy as an outpatient. One of Mr. Davis's goals is to regain his "normal" activity level. Mr. Davis's physical therapist supports this goal and selects the 6MWD as one outcome measure that will be used to determine his progress. Mr. Davis weighs 70 kg and his height is 172 cm. Applying the reference equation for men, the physical therapist sets Mr. Davis's target 6MWD at 594 m.

Single-Group Percentile Method: What Is It?

This method is similar to the percentile improvement method (PIM) described in the preceding chapter. However, rather than being interested in the change necessary to achieve a true or important improvement, the focus is now on a measure's target value that represents the desired outcome. This approach is based on the notion that if there is a reasonably good chance a patient's value on a measure is consistent with the values of patients who report a satisfactory outcome, then a patient with a value in this range has achieved a satisfactory outcome.

Study Design

A cohort of patients with the condition and characteristics of interest is assessed following a course of treatment. From the original cohort, a reference standard is used to identify a subsample of patients who have achieved a satisfactory outcome.

How Percentile Values Are Calculated

Following the example for the PIM method, the investigator selects an arbitrary percentile rank that will be used to identify the threshold score on the measure for a satisfactory outcome. Unlike the PIM analysis where all improvement scores were considered positive, the scale orientation comes into play when considering the target outcome score for a measure. For some outcome measures a lower score represents a favorable outcome (e.g., many pain scales), whereas for other measures a higher score signifies a favorable outcome (e.g., 20-m walk pace). For measures where lower scores represent a favorable outcome, higher percentile values are selected to identify the threshold outcome score. Outcome measure scores equal to or less than the threshold value represent satisfactory outcome scores. Figure 7-1 provides an example using the 80th percentile applied to the 0- to 10-point numeric pain rating scale. This example contains the post-treatment pain scores for 100 hypothetical patients deemed to have had a satisfactory outcome. These data can also be summarized as a cumulative distribution plot, an example of which is shown in Figure 7-2. Cumulative distribution graphs represent an efficient and flexible way of matching a percentile value to a measure's target value.[8] Regardless of the graphing technique applied, we see that both methods identify a pain score of 2 or less as representing a satisfactory outcome for these hypothetical patients.

In contrast, Figures 7-3 and 7-4 show the application of the 20th percentile as the threshold value for the 20-m walk pace where higher values represent more positive outcomes. This

Text continued on page 112

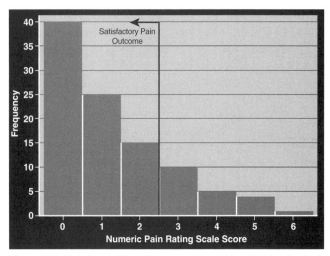

Figure 7-1 Satisfactory Pain Outcomes Scores Identified by the 80th Percentile

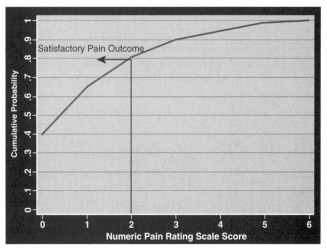

Figure 7-2 Satisfactory Pain Outcomes Scores Identified by the 80th Percentile

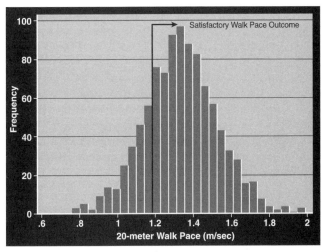

Figure 7-3 Satisfactory 20-m Walking Speeds Identified by the 80th Percentile

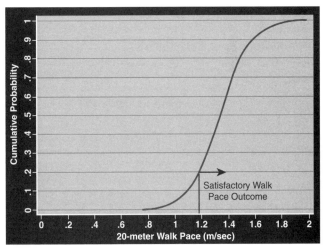

Figure 7-4 Satisfactory 20-m Walking Speeds Identified by the 20th Percentile

example displays 20-m walking speeds of 1,000 hypothetical patients with OA of the knee deemed to have achieved a satisfactory outcome. In this case, walking speeds equal to or greater than the 20th percentile distance represent a satisfactory outcome. Figure 7-4 displays the same data as a cumulative distribution plot.

The only assumption required for this analysis is that patients contributing data have achieved a satisfactory outcome. Because the threshold value for a satisfactory outcome is based on a percentile rank, the distribution of outcome scores need not be consistent with a normal distribution.

Interpretation

The interpretation is that patients meeting or exceeding the threshold value (either positive or negative, depending on the scale orientation) have achieved a satisfactory outcome.

The Bottom Line

This method shares the same limitation as the percentile method applied to PIM described in the previous chapter. Specifically, the results are reported with respect to patients known to have achieved a satisfactory outcome. In clinical practice a patient presents with a measured value and the physical therapist must decide whether it is more likely to be associated with patients who have achieved a satisfactory outcome or those who have not.

A Clinical Example **What the Researcher Did**

This example is based on the work of Tubach et al, who conducted a study to determine the Patient Acceptable Symptom State (PASS) of pain for patients with osteoarthritis of the hip or knee.[8] The PASS is defined as "the value beyond which patients can consider themselves well."[8] We consider this value to represent a satisfactory outcome and equate it to the target goal score. Tubach et al followed a group of patients for 4 weeks, during which time they received treatment. Patients completed a 100-mm visual analog scale at the beginning and end of the 4-week period. At the 4-week assessment, patients also answered the question "Taking into account all the activities you have during your daily life, your level of pain, and also your functional impairment, do you consider that your current state is satisfactory?" Patients responding "yes" to this question composed the sample used to calculate the PASS score. Keeping in mind that lower pain scores are associated with better outcomes, the investigators equated the PASS pain score with the 75th percentile. PASS pain scores for the hip and knee were 35 mm and 32 mm, respectively.

How the Physical Therapist Applied the Information

Ms. O'Maly, a patient with osteoarthritis of the right knee, reported a pain score of 63 mm at her initial visit. Being familiar with the study presented above, Ms. O'Maly's physical therapist formed the following goal: "To decrease Ms. O'Maly's pain score to 30 mm or fewer in 4 weeks." At the 4-week follow-up visit, Ms. O'Maly reported a pain score of 21 mm and she was discharged from active treatment with a home program.

▶ Diagnostic Test Methodology

In the previous chapter we described how diagnostic test methodology (DTM) is applied in the context of identifying important or true change scores. In this chapter we show how DTM is used to identify the target goal value.

What Is It?

Applied in the current context, DTM aims at identifying a threshold value that maximizes the correct classification of patients as having met their target goal state or not.

Study Design

With two exceptions the study design is identical to that described in the previous chapter. The first exception is that the reference standard labels patients as having achieved their target state or not. The second difference is that the identified value is for a measure's score rather than a change score. Figure 7-5 shows a sample 2 × 2 table appropriately labeled for identifying a target state value.

		Reference Standard Satisfactory Outcome Achieved		
		Yes	No	
Outcome Measure Interpretation	Satisfactory Outcome Yes	a	b	a + b
	Satisfactory Outcome No	c	d	c + d
		a + c	b + d	n = a + b + c + d

Figure 7-5 Illustration of a 2 × 2 Table Used to Summarize the Results from a Diagnostic Test Target State Study

How Receiver Operating Characteristic Curves Are Constructed

The target goal value is defined as the value that jointly maximizes sensitivity and specificity. (See DTM in the previous chapter for a detailed description of this analytic method.)

Assumptions for DTM to Be Valid

The only assumption is that the reference standard accurately classifies patients as having achieved a satisfactory outcome or not. The distributions of the measure's scores for patients meeting or not meeting their target state need not be normally distributed.

Interpretation

Patients with outcome measure values equal to or better than the identified satisfactory outcome value are considered to have met their goals.

The Bottom Line

Because DTM provides information concerning patients who have or have not achieved a satisfactory outcome, we consider this methodology to be superior to single-group designs such as the PIM. Moreover, DTM allows the calculation of predictive values, and it is these values that provide physical therapists with the chance of correctly labeling patients as having achieved their goals.

| A Clinical Example | ## What the Researcher Did

This example is based on the work of Kamper et al.[9] The goal of their study was to identify a Roland-Morris questionnaire (RMQ) score that maximized the correct classification of patients with low-back pain as being completely recovered. The RMQ is a 24-item self-report measure of pain-related disability. Items are scored "1" if endorsed by a patient and "0" if not endorsed. Accordingly, total RMQ scores can vary from 0 to 24, with higher scores representing greater amounts of pain-related disability. The RMQ and a global perceived effect scale—which acted as the reference standard—were administered following a course of treatment. An ROC curve analysis was constructed and a RMQ score of 2 or less was found to represent the threshold for "completely recovered." The area under the ROC curve was 0.85 and the sensitivity and specificity associated with a RMQ score of 2 were approximately 82% and 79%, respectively. Assuming that a patient's pretest chance of meeting the target goal is 50%, and applying the reported sensitivity and specificity values, the corresponding positive and negative predictive values are 80% and 81%, respectively (see Fig. 7-6).

		True State Satisfactory Outcome Achieved		
		Yes	No	
Outcome Measure Interpretation	≤2	82	21	103
	>2	18	79	97
		100	100	200

Figure 7-6 Table Illustrating Results for a Sensitivity of 82%, Specificity of 79%, and Pretest Chance of Meeting the Target State of 50%

How the Physical Therapist Applied the Information

Mr. MacIntyre, a patient with low-back pain, reported a RMQ score of 12/24 at his initial assessment. Being familiar with the study reported above, Mr. MacIntyre's physical therapist formed the following measurable target state goal: "To decrease Mr. MacIntyre's RMQ score to 2 or less points in 3 weeks." At the 3-week follow-up assessment, Mr. MacIntyre's RMQ score was 5/24. Given that the negative predictive value is 81%, the physical therapist concluded with a high level of confidence that Mr. MacIntyre had not yet met his target state value and treatment was continued.

Chapter Summary

- Long-term measurable goals are typically written in terms of a target value.
- When identifying a target value for a patient it is essential that the reference sample has characteristics similar to the patient of interest.
- Normal-value tables may be useful when full recovery is expected; however, from a practical perspective they can account for only a few potential predictor variables (often just age and gender) and estimates may lack specificity for many patients.
- Provided the sample size is sufficiently large and representative, reference equations have the potential to provide a target value that takes into consideration a greater number of patient characteristics than can be reported in normal-value tables.
- Provided the reference sample is representative of patients with characteristics similar to the patient of interest, reference equations can also be used to model target values for persons not expected to meet value of the typical "healthy" age- and gender-matched person.
- When applying the percentile approach, the choice of percentile defining the target value is arbitrary and dependent on the scale orientation.
- DTM provides an estimate of the target value that maximizes the correct classification of patients as having met or not met their goal.

- Only predictive values obtained from DTM offer the chance of correctly labeling patients as having met their goals or not.

■ Reference List

1. Sackett DL. Evidence-based medicine. *Semin Perinatol* 1997;21:3–5.

2. Petersen P, Petrick M, Connor H, Conklin D. Grip strength and hand dominance: Challenging the 10% rule. *Am J Occup Ther* 1989;43:444–7.

3. Shultz SJ, Nguyen AD. Bilateral asymmetries in clinical measures of lower-extremity anatomic characteristics. *Clin J Sport Med* 2007;17:357–61.

4. Ware JEJ, Sherbourne CD. The MOS 36-item short-form health survey (SF-36). I. Conceptual framework and item selection. *Med Care* 1992;30:473–83.

5. Hopman WM, Towheed T, Anastassiades T, Tenenhouse A, Poliquin S, Berger C, et al. Canadian normative data for the SF-36 health survey. Canadian Multicentre Osteoporosis Study Research Group. *Cmaj* 2000;163:265–71.

6. Kleinbaum DG, Kupper LL, Nizam A, Muller KE. *Applied Regression Analysis and Other Multivariable Methods*, 4th ed. Boston, MA: Duxbury; 2008.

7. Enright PL, Sherrill DL. Reference equations for the six-minute walk in healthy adults. *Am J Respir Crit Care Med* 1998;158:1384–7.

8. Tubach F, Ravaud P, Baron G, Falissard B, Logeart I, Bellamy N, et al. Evaluation of clinically relevant changes in patient reported outcomes in knee and hip osteoarthritis: The minimal clinically important improvement. *Ann Rheum Dis* 2005;64:29–33.

9. Steffen TM, Hacker TA, Mollinger L. Age- and gender-related test performance in community-dwelling elderly people: Six-Minute Walk Test, Berg Balance Scale, Timed Up & Go Test, and gait speeds. *Phys Ther* 2002;82:128–37.

Chapter 8

When Should Reassessments Take Place?

■ *Two components of a measurable goal are the target value and the expected time frame for meeting the target value. We learned in previous chapters that the target value can be written in terms of a change score or as an absolute value for the outcome of interest. Having found prognostic evidence regarding your patient's condition, the trick now is to place a time estimate on when you think the patient might expect to experience an appreciable change in his or her condition. Our take is that there is less evidence to guide decisions regarding temporal elements of goals than even the goals themselves. We have come up with two approaches that may help you in deciding on the optimal time frames for reevaluating your patients to assess for progression toward goal attainment.*

What's Ahead

In this chapter we describe two methods for identifying the anticipated time frame for meeting a goal. We also introduce the important concept that ignoring the ideal reassessment interval will increase the error rate in determining whether patients have met their goal values.

The Concept Behind This Question

Determining optimal reassessment intervals requires knowledge of the expected change profile for patients similar to the patient of interest and a measurement strategy that maximizes the accuracy of clinical decisions formed at the time of reassessment. There are two important concepts embedded in this statement.

The first idea is that change profiles exist for specific conditions and patient characteristics and that this evidence can be found in the literature. The second thought is that optimal reassessment intervals exist and that these intervals will vary depending on where a patient is with respect to the clinical course of the condition. By change profile, we mean how a patient's value on the outcome of interest changes over time. Included in this concept are both the expected rate of change and the absolute values of the outcome measure at all points in time over the clinical course of a condition. The second concept acknowledges that specifying the appropriate reassessment interval will enhance the accuracy of determining whether a goal has been met or not. We show that reassessments can be most efficient if they are done at a time when expected changes are optimally estimated. Your time is valuable and reassessments take time. Completing reassessments at optimal points in time during the plan of care makes most efficient use of the time you have to reassess your patients.

▶ Methods Used to Determine Target Goal Values

Modeling Change Over Time: Growth Curves: What Is It?

This approach seeks to identify a change profile for patients who have conditions and characteristics that are similar to those of your patient. The profile is usually expressed as an equation (growth model) and as a pictorial representation that graphs the outcome measure value on the *y*-axis against the number of weeks after a common time point (e.g., onset of the condition or days post-surgery) on the *x*-axis.

Study Design

Growth curves are developed from a longitudinal study design where multiple measurements are obtained on patients with the condition of interest. The timing of the measurement and the number of measurements need not be the same for all patients.

In fact, obtaining measurements at different time points for different patients allows for the modeling of a smoother growth curve than had measurements been taken at the same time points for all patients.

How Growth Curves Are Constructed

The first step a researcher takes when modeling a growth curve is to plot the outcome measure values against the number of days after a common time point. For the rest of this discussion we assume the common time point is the day of surgery for a total knee arthroplasty (TKA). The second step is to interpret the plotted data and select a mathematical model that is likely to best describe the relationship between the outcome measure values and the days post-TKA. For many conditions seen by physical therapists change occurs rapidly during the first several encounters or weeks and then progresses more slowly until the target value (plateau on graph) is reached.[1-4] Figure 8-1 shows modeled

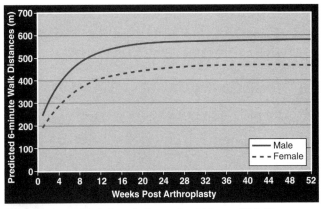

Figure 8-1 Modeled Growth Curves for 6-Minute Walk Test Distances for Men and Women Post-Total Knee Arthroplasty.[3] Adapted from Kennedy DM, Stratford PW, Riddle DL, Hanna SE, Gollish JD. Assessing recovery and establishing prognosis following total knee arthroplasty. *Phys Ther* 2008;88:22–32. Reprinted with permission.

6-minute walk distance (6MWD) growth curves adapted from the work of Kennedy et al for men and women post-TKA.[3]

Several requirements are necessary for this approach to be useful. First, it is crucial that the patient sample is representative of the condition and patient characteristics of interest. Also, the sample must be large enough to provide confidence in outcome values predicted by the model. A second assumption is that study data are missing at random. This means that a missing value—that is, the value a patient would have had if a measurement were taken at a time point—is not due to the value the patient would have provided had a measurement been performed at that time point. For example, a patient who did not attend an evaluation session because his functional status prevented him from coming would not be considered missing at random. However, a patient who did not attend because of a snowstorm or flat tire would be considered missing at random.

Interpretation

Although growth curves are based on mathematical models that at times can appear quite complex, the growth curve itself is easily interpreted. Quite simply, the curve provides a time-specific estimate of the outcome measure value for the typical patient with the condition and characteristics of interest. Referring to Figure 8-1, the typical female patient 12 weeks post-TKA would be expected to have a 6MWD of approximately 410 m.

The Bottom Line

Growth curves provide an ideal way of describing the expected clinical course of the typical patient. In addition, they are essential for specifying the optimal interval between assessments when specifying measurable goals. One limitation is that we don't have a large number of growth curves for the conditions seen by physical therapists, but we expect that more researchers will see the value of this approach and report growth curves for more conditions.

| A Clinical Example | **What the Researcher Did**

This example is based on the study by Kennedy et al, who investigated 84 patients post-TKA secondary to osteoarthritis. These investigators collected 6MWD data for up to 60 weeks post-TKA and determined the growth curves for both men and women. Forty patients were men and their median age and BMI were 67 years and 29 kg/m^2, respectively. The investigators found the following nonlinear model best fit the data for men:[3]

6MWD (m) = 577.7 + (185.7 − 577.7)
    × exponent(−exponent(−1.7) × weeks post arthroplasty)

The growth curve associated with this model is shown in Figure 8-1.

How a Physical Therapist Could Apply the Information

Mr. Burns, a 65 year old with a BMI of 30 kg/m^2, underwent a TKA 2 weeks ago. At today's assessment, his 6MWD is 294 m. Using Mr. Burns's current 6MWD as a baseline, his physical therapist set one short-term and one long-term target goal. The short-term goal was "to increase Mr. Burns's 6MWD by 62 m in 2 weeks." The long-term or target goal was "to increase Mr. Burns's 6MWD to 577 m at 22 weeks post-TKA."

To form the short-term goal, the physical therapist had first to determine a value that likely represented a true change in 6MWD. A literature search identified an article that estimated the minimal detectable change at a 90% confidence level (MDC$_{90}$) to be approximately 62 m in patients with osteoarthritis.[5] Using the growth curve, the physical therapist identified the interval over which the typical patient with a 2-week 6MWD of 294 m would improve by 62 m. Notice that as the time post-TKA increases, the interval necessary to achieve a change of 62 m also increases. To identify the target value and when it would likely be attained, the physical therapist again referred to the growth curve. The curve plateaus at approximately 22 weeks, yielding a value of about 577 m (i.e., the limit value). Accordingly, the stated target goal was "to increase Mr. Burns's 6MWD to 577 m in 20 weeks."

Although choosing a literature-based value that is likely to represent a true change (e.g., MDC$_{90}$) may seem natural, the consequence of misjudging the appropriate time frame for achieving the goal value is less obvious and may seem trivial. In fact, often it is customary to schedule reassessments at regular and evenly spaced intervals. Later in this chapter we show that scheduling reassessments at the optimal time points will minimize mislabeling patients as having changed or not.

Compilation of Information from Separate Studies: What Is it?

Although studies reporting growth curves are most informative, at the time of writing this text few examples were available for outcomes of interest to physical therapists. A second, less rigorous approach is to construct a "growth curve" from the results of multiple studies that describe the values of the measurement of interest over varying time periods. When applying this method it is important that the patient characteristics and other clinical circumstances (e.g., type of surgery, intervention, etc.) are similar across studies, as well as to the patients and conditions to which you will apply the results.

Approach for Constructing a Growth Curve

The first step is for the interested physical therapist or, better yet, a like-minded group of therapists to seek out relevant studies reported in the literature. Ideally, the patient characteristics and conditions of measurement in these studies should be similar to the target group of patients. Once a number of studies have been identified, the next step is to summarize and plot the data with the outcome measure's values on the *y*-axis and the number of weeks after the common time point on the *x*-axis.

Interpretation

The interpretation of the findings is similar to that described for growth curves.

The Bottom Line

This method provides a practical approach for estimating the expected progress of patients with the condition and characteristics of interest.

Table 8-1	Knee Flexion Range-of-Motion Values at Specific Time Points Post-Total Knee Arthroplasty

Approximate Weeks Post-Arthroplasty

Source	1	4	6	8	12	26	52
Kumar[8]	84°		104°		113°		
Mizner[9]		94°		109°	114°	116°	
Lombardi[10]			110°				
Petterson[11]					115°		119°
Kramer[12]					100°		105°
Ritter[13]							
Males						113°	115°
Females						110°	113°
Average	84°	94°	107°	109°	110.5°	113°	113°

A Clinical Example	**What the Physical Therapist Did**

A physical therapy department that specializes in the treatment of patients receiving TKA was interested in finding information that would assist in forming measurable goals for knee flexion range of motion (ROM) post-arthroplasty. Unable to find a study that modeled ROM post-TKA, the department conducted a literature search to identify studies that reported knee flexion ROM at various time points post-TKA. Six studies were identified, the results of which are summarized in Table 8-1.

Figure 8-2 shows the results graphically, including a smoothed curve (bold) representing the average of the week-specific results.

How the Physical Therapist Applied the Information

Mrs. Brown received a TKA 4 weeks ago. Today, her knee flexion ROM is 98°. Mrs. Brown's physical therapist was aware of a study that estimated a detectable change in knee flexion ROM to be 9°.[4] Using this information and the derived growth curve (Fig. 8-2), the physical therapist set the following short- and long-term goals: "To increase Mrs. Brown's knee flexion range by 9° in 4 weeks; to increase Mrs. Brown's knee flexion range to 113° by 26 weeks post-arthroplasty."

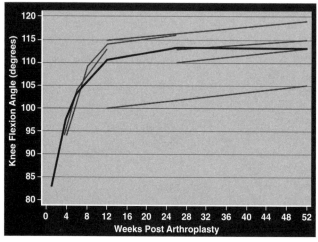

Figure 8-2 Modeled Growth Curve (bold line) Based on Results from Six Studies

▶ Rationale for an Optimal Reassessment Interval

Two components of a measurable goal are the target value and time frame for achieving the target value. The target value can be written as a change (e.g., to increase the 6MWT distance by 62 m) or as an absolute value (e.g., to increase the 6MWT distance to 577 m). In the first section of this chapter, we reviewed two methods for establishing the expected clinical course of a patient. The aim of each method was to construct a growth curve that displayed the clinical course of a typical patient. In each example the physical therapist combined information from the growth curve with knowledge of the threshold value for improvement to determine the reassessment interval.

In contrast to this information-driven approach to determine the reassessment interval, sound practice has often encouraged frequent reassessments, particularly when the outcome measures are easy to administer, such as ROM and single-item ratings scales. We now look at the consequence of reassessing patients sooner or later than would be suggested by the information-driven approach.

In Chapter 6 we learned that assessing change could be conceptualized as diagnosing change. Applied in this context, the diagnosed condition is true or important change, rather than the presence or absence of a disease. We also learned that the positive predictive value provides the chance that a patient has improved given a positive test result (i.e., a change score equal to or greater than the threshold improvement value) and that the negative predictive value provides the chance that a patient has not improved given a negative test result (i.e., a change score less than the threshold improvement value). An important concept when interpreting predictive values is the realization that they are dependent on prevalence or pretest chance of improvement. By this we mean the chance a physical therapist assigns to a patient as having improved prior to the interpretation of the outcome measure result. As the pretest chance of improvement increases, the positive predictive value increases and the negative predictive value decreases. As the pretest chance of improvement decreases, the negative predictive value increases and the positive predictive value decreases.

So how does this affect the selection of a reassessment interval? Recall that a growth curve provides the expected change for the typical or average patient with the characteristics of interest. Stated another way, 50% of patients would be expected to improve more than the exact growth curve value and 50% of patients would be expected to improve less than the exact growth curve value. When the reassessment interval is set to when the typical patient would be expected to improve by the threshold amount, the physical therapist is setting the pretest chance of improvement to 50%.[6] Shortening the reassessment interval reduces the percentage of patients expected to improve and consequently the pretest chance of improvement; increasing the reassessment interval increases the number of patients expected to improve and the pretest chance of improvement. We now look at the consequences of shortening and lengthening the reassessment interval.

A Clinical Example | **Impact of Reassessment Interval**

This example draws on the work of Cleland et al, who applied diagnostic test methodology to estimate the minimal clinically important improvement (MCII) value for the 11-point numeric pain rating scale (0 no pain, 10 worst pain imaginable) when applied to patients with neck pain.[7] These investigators reported an area under the receiver operating characteristic (ROC) curve to be 0.85. They found that a reduction in pain of 1.3 points maximized the correct classification of patients as having improved an important amount. The corresponding sensitivity and specificity values for this improvement score were 0.88 and 0.71, respectively.

Using these sensitivity and specificity values, we now show the impact on the predictive values of assessing patients for three pretest conditions. The first condition applies the reassessment before the typical patient is expected to achieve an improvement equal to the MCII. For this example we assign a pretest chance of achieving an important improvement of 20%. For the second condition we assign a 50% chance of achieving a MCII. This corresponds to the ideal reassessment interval. The third condition extends the reassessment interval beyond that of when the typical patient is expected to achieve a MCII. We assign an 80% pretest chance of achieving a MCII for this reassessment interval.

Referring to Table 8-2, we see that the misclassification percentage, as characterized by the sum of false-positive and false-negative percentages, is minimized at 39% for a pretest chance of achieving a MCII of 50%. Scheduling the reassessment too early increases the misclassification percentage (61%), principally due to an increase in the false-positive percentage. Extending the reassessment interval beyond the ideal reassessment interval also increases the misclassification percent (48%); however, this time it's the false-negative percentage that accounts for most of the misclassifications. In summary, a consequence of scheduling a reassessment too early will be to mislabel an increased number of patients as having improved when in truth they have not. Conversely, a consequence of scheduling a reassessment too late will be to label an increased number of patients as having not improved when in fact that have truly improved.

Table 8-2 Impact of Reassessment Interval on the Accuracy of Correctly Classifying a Patient Based on the Estimated Minimal Clinically Important Improvement Value

| | Pretest Chance of Correctly Classifying a Patient | | |
	20% (Too early)	50% (Just right)	80% (Too late)
Positive predictive value (%)	43%	75%	92%
False positive (%)	57%	25%	8%
Negative predictive value (%)	96%	86%	60%
False negative (%)	4%	14%	40%
Misclassification (%)	61%	39%	48%

Chapter Summary

- Two components of a measurable goal are the goal value and the expected time frame for meeting the goal value.
- Growth curves provide a simple yet effective way of conveying time-specific outcome measure values, expected rates of change in outcome, and the long-term target value.
- Formal growth curve analyses are derived from mathematical models.
- Information from mathematical models of growth curves can be presented in an easily interpreted graph that plots the outcome measure value on the *y*-axis against the time after a common event on the *x*-axis.
- Growth curves can be "informally" constructed by combining information from multiple studies, provided the patient characteristics and conditions of measurement are similar across studies.
- The optimal reassessment interval is when 50% of patients with characteristics similar to the patient of interest would be expected to meet the goal value.

▪ Reference List

1. Palisano RJ, Hanna SE, Rosenbaum PL, Russell DJ, Walter SD, Wood EP, et al. Validation of a model of gross motor function for children with cerebral palsy. *Phys Ther* 2000;80:974–85.

2. Oberg T, Karsznia A, Oberg K. Basic gait parameters: Reference data for normal subjects, 10–79 years of age. *J Rehab Res and Develop* 1993;30: 210–23.

3. Kennedy DM, Stratford PW, Riddle DL, Hanna SE, Gollish JD. Assessing recovery and establishing prognosis following total knee arthroplasty. *Phys Ther* 2008;88:22–32.

4. Stratford PW, Kennedy DM, Robarts SF. Modelling knee range of motion post arthroplasty: Clinical applications. *Physiother Can* 2010;62:378–87.

5. Kennedy DM, Stratford PW, Wessel J, Gollish JD, Penney D. Assessing stability and change of four performance measures: A longitudinal study evaluating outcome following total hip and knee arthroplasty. *BMC Musculoskelet Disord* 2005;6:3.

6. Stratford PW. Diagnosing patient change: Impact of reassessment interval. *Physiother Can* 2000;52:225–8.

7. Tousignant M, Poulin L, Marchand S, Viau A, Place C. The Modified-Modified Schober Test for range of motion assessment of lumbar flexion in patients with low back pain: A study of criterion validity, intra- and inter-rater reliability and minimum metrically detectable change. *Disabil and Rehab* 2005;27:553–9.

8. Kumar PJ, McPherson EJ, Dorr LD, Wan Z, Baldwin K. Rehabilitation after total knee arthroplasty: A comparison of 2 rehabilitation techniques. *Clin Orthop Relat Res* 1996:93–101.

9. Mizner RL, Petterson SC, Snyder-Mackler L. Quadriceps strength and the time course of functional recovery after total knee arthroplasty. *J Orthop Sports Phys Ther* 2005;35:424–36.

10. Lombardi AV, Jr., Berend KR, Walter CA, Aziz-Jacobo J, Cheney NA. Is recovery faster for mobile-bearing unicompartmental than total knee arthroplasty? *Clin Orthop Relat Res* 2009;467: 1450–7.

11. Petterson SC, Mizner RL, Stevens JE, Raisis L, Bodenstab A, Newcomb W, et al. Improved function from progressive strengthening interventions after total knee arthroplasty: A randomized clinical trial with an imbedded prospective cohort. *Arthritis Rheum* 2009; 61:174–83.

12. Kramer JF, Speechley M, Bourne R, Rorabeck C, Vaz M. Comparison of clinic- and home-based rehabilitation programs after total knee arthroplasty. *Clin Orthop Relat Res* 2003:225–34.

13. Ritter MA, Wing JT, Berend ME, Davis KE, Meding JB. The clinical effect of gender on outcome of total knee arthroplasty. *J Arthroplasty* 2008;23:331–6.

Chapter 9

Acknowledging Barriers and Identifying Barrier-Busting Strategies

▪ *Choosing a standardized outcome measure that will be effective in your clinical setting can be challenging and requires some work on the front end to help ensure success. All too often, physical therapists enthusiastic about using standardized outcome measures in their practices have become jaded when attempting to implement the measures. This has often led to abandoning them. There are two prominent reasons for this. The first is that the physical therapists did not have a clear vision of what they wanted to assess with the measure. The second reason is that the therapists did not consider potential barriers associated with implementing the selected outcome measure in the therapists' unique clinical settings. In this chapter we first identify potential barriers to the successful implementation of outcome measures in clinical practice and then offer six steps that will enhance your chance of selecting a measure that can be successfully implemented in your clinical setting.*

❱ Barriers to the Successful Implementation of Outcome Measures in Clinical Practice

It may seem rather strange to devote a section of this text to barriers associated with implementing outcome measures in clinical practice. After all, aren't we proponents of standardized outcome measures? However, without acknowledging and addressing these barriers, the chance of successfully implementing standardized measures in busy practice settings is greatly reduced.

A number of published reports have consistently identified these potential barriers.[1–4] In some instances, the rationale for a barrier is real; in other cases, the reasoning for a barrier is perceived or unfounded. In this section we identify frequently reported barriers under the following headings: (1) "Barriers Affecting the Therapist," (2) "Barriers Affecting the Patient-Measure Interaction," and (3) "Resource and Organizational Barriers." This is followed by the introduction of six strategies that will facilitate the successful implementation of standardized outcome measures in your practice. We call these barrier-busting strategies.

Barriers Affecting the Therapist

1. "I'm really doing this for someone else, and that someone else is not my patient." Often, the use of standardized outcome measures have been thrust on therapists by administrators, payers, or professional bodies. Consequently, there is a perception that the extra time and effort put into administrating and scoring the measure is for someone else, and little is to be gained by the therapist or patient. To overcome this barrier, the added value of applying "yet another" test or measure must be made obvious.

2. "I can infer activity limitations and participation restrictions with a high degree of confidence from impairment measures that I currently apply." Several mistaken beliefs contribute to this barrier. The first misconception is that a high correlation exists among impairments (e.g., range of motion and strength), activities (e.g., walking and stairs), and participatory endeavors (e.g., working and recreational pursuits). This is not the case in most instances. Typical correlations between impairments and activities lie

in the range of 0.20 to 0.60.[5–6] A correlation of 0.60 indicates that knowing the information obtained from the impairment allows one to predict about 36% of the information concerning the activity. Clearly, this is not a great deal. The second assumption is that change takes place in a linear and orderly manner. That is, a change in impairment results in a change in activity that in turn leads to a change in participation. Combined, these beliefs foster the notion that because impairments are routinely assessed, there is no need to apply additional measures that evaluate activities and participatory endeavors directly. Awareness of the modest relationship among different outcomes is necessary to overcome this barrier.

3. "I do not understand what a measure's score means." This barrier addresses the interpretability of a score or change score provided by the measure. We have learned previously in Chapter 5 that interpretability considers the extent to which one can assign qualitative meaning to quantitative scores.[7] For a measure to be useful, it must contribute additional clinically relevant information.

4. "I have insufficient time to administer and score the measure." This barrier can be either real or perceived. An important question to answer is "How much time are you willing to spend to gain additional clinically useful information?"

5. "I do not have the necessary skills to seek out and evaluate potentially useful measures." This barrier is real, and one goal of this text is to provide readers with skills necessary to locate and appraise outcome measures. These skills are introduced in Chapter 10.

6. "The existing measures are not applicable for my patient." The essence of this barrier is that a standardized outcome measure does not exist for the attribute, condition, or circumstance of interest. This barrier arises for two reasons. First, to truly know that a relevant

measure does not exist, one must be proficient at searching and evaluating the literature (see Chapter 10 for help with this). Increasing one's skill level in these areas is likely to show that in many instances relevant measures do exist. The second reason for this belief is that often therapists are "locked in" to looking for a disease- or condition-specific measure. When an appropriate condition- or disease-specific measure cannot be found, an alternate solution is to consider a standardized patient-specific measure.

Barriers Affecting the Patient-Measure Interaction

1. "The measure places too much burden on the patient." Although some measures may have excellent measurement properties, they may be too long to be completed by many patients. It is essential to match the measure to your patient and clinical environment.

2. "The measure's difficulty level is not appropriate for the patient." This barrier differs from the previous one in that it is not the time required to complete the measure that is the problem, but rather it is that the measure is either too difficult or too easy to gain an accurate impression of the patient's ability. For example, a test that assesses the time required to walk 400 m would be inappropriate for patients who are incapable of walking this distance. This test would also be inappropriate to assess the functional recovery of a high-performance athlete whose problem presents only after running several kilometers over hilly terrain. Once again, the solution is to match the measure to your patient.

3. "The patient cannot comprehend the measure." This barrier is particularly relevant for self-report measures and it may present in two ways. First, if the measure has been validated in one language (e.g., English) and many of your patients are not fluent in this language,

then the measure cannot be applied with confidence to these patients. This barrier can be overcome by seeking out measures that have been validated for languages relevant to your patient population. A second consideration is the extent to which the vocabulary used in the questionnaire is consistent with the typical vocabulary and reading level of your patients. Here the patient understands the language of the self-report measure (i.e., the questionnaire is written in English and the patient comprehends English); however, many of the words and phrases used are unfamiliar to the patient. It is often recommended that questionnaires should be written for the reading level of a 12 year old.[8]

Resource and Organizational Barriers

1. "The measure requires special equipment or skills." Some measures are expensive to acquire and implement. The cost may be associated with purchasing the necessary equipment, obtaining copyright permission, paying a user fee, or learning the skills necessary to administer and score the measure. It is essential to identify these costs. Measures that are too costly should be ruled out.

2. "The measure is never in my hands when I need it." This barrier is frequently encountered once a measure has been chosen. To be a useful clinical decision-making aid, a measure must be available to the patient-therapist interaction at key decision points. These decision points include the initial assessment, relevant follow-up assessments as specified by measurable goals, and the discharge assessment. To facilitate their appropriate use, outcome measures must be readily accessible to the therapist.

3. "It is difficult to keep track of all the measurements when multiple outcomes are being assessed." Because all outcomes of interest for a patient rarely change at the same rate, there will be times when the outcomes will be assessed at different occasions. Even though all the

information is recorded in a patient's chart, it may take considerable time to locate and synthesize the relevant information. There are too many pieces of paper and too many notes found in different locations of the medical record. It is vital that the necessary information is easily accessible at key decision points over the course of treatment.

▷ Finding the Best Measures for You: Six Barrier-Busting Steps

Step 1.   *Start by declaring what it is you hope to assess with the measure.* It is essential to have a clear vision of what you intend to measure. To solidify this vision, we advocate constructing a carefully written statement detailing what you wish to measure. A well-written statement is invaluable when you search for a measure. Two examples are as follows:

- I wish to identify a standardized self-report measure of pain-related functional status that is sensitive to changes typically seen in outpatients presenting with acute, subacute, and chronic low-back pain, and who are treated with interventions applied by physical therapists.
- I wish to identify a standardized performance measure that assesses lower extremity functional status and is sensitive to change in persons with Parkinson disease.

Step 2.   *State important patient-related constraints.* Important considerations include the patient burden, the appropriate difficulty level, and whether the measure is presented in a format that can be comprehended by the patient.

- Many patients with low-back pain seen in my clinic speak and read Spanish. Therefore, I wish to identify a standardized self-report measure of back-pain-related functional status that has been validated in Spanish and English.

Step 3. *State important constraints relevant to your clinical setting.* Not only is it essential to have a clear vision of what you intend to measure, it is equally important to consider the feasibility of implementing the measure in your practice.

- Declare the amount of therapist-patient interaction time you are willing to spend acquiring additional clinically useful information and how much time you are willing to spend scoring the measure. For example, I am willing to spend 3 minutes more with the patient to acquire additional information, and I am willing to spend 30 seconds scoring the measure, provided computational aids (e.g., a calculator or computer) are not required.
- State the extent to which you are willing to "purchase" additional resources required to implement the outcome measure in your clinical setting. The "purchase" may be the cost of the measure, additional equipment necessary to support the measure (e.g., a computer or software), or the hours of your time required to learn how to apply and score the measure. For example, I am not willing to spend money purchasing a measure or equipment; however, I am willing to devote 3 hours of self-study time to learn how to use the measure.

Step 4. *Search effectively and efficiently for relevant outcome measures.* Locating a measure to meet your needs requires a proficient search strategy. Several starting points are listed below. Detailed search strategies are discussed in Chapter 10.

- Peruse outcome measure databases (online and textbooks).
- Try a Google Scholar search.
- Conduct a literature search (e.g., PubMed, CINAHL).
- Examine the reference lists from publications obtained from your primary literature search.

Step 5. *Seek out measures that provide information on the interpretation of score values.* The primary reason for implementing an additional measure is to acquire clinically useful information that is not being obtained from currently applied measures. If an outcome measure's scores do not have meaning, this goal cannot be met. For this reason we recommend that if information concerning the interpretation of score values is not available, look for another measure. Here are several questions to consider when judging the extent to which information exists concerning the interpretation of score values.

• Does information exist concerning measurement error?
• Does information exist for normal or customary values for the patients/condition of interest?
• Does information exist for what constitutes a true or clinically important change?
• Does information exist concerning the expected terminal or target value and when it is likely to be achieved?
• Does information exist concerning the expected rate of change?

The answers to these questions are essential if one is to write meaningful, measurable goals and judge the extent to which a patient is "on track" during the course of treatment.

Step 6. *Scrutinize the measurement properties of the measure relevant to your clinical context.* Two important points require consideration. The first acknowledges the relevant measurement properties for an outcome measure, and the second stresses that measurement properties exist in a context.

• Outcome measures are used to assess the status of patients at a point in time and to evaluate change over time. Accordingly, the measurement properties of interest are reliability, cross-sectional validity, and longitudinal validity. Cross-sectional validity assesses the extent to which a measure assesses what it is intended to measure at a point in time. Longitudinal validity comments on a measure's ability to detect true change in the characteristic of interest. The terms *sensitivity to change* and *responsiveness* are often used interchangeably with the term *longitudinal validity*.

- The second consideration is that measurements take place in a context. The context may be a condition (e.g., osteoarthritis of the knee, sprained ankle), a clinical setting, or a unique set of patient circumstances. Stated another way, measures do not have measurement properties—measurement scores do.[9] The important point is that the measurement properties obtained for a measure in one context (e.g., 6-minute walk distance for patients with respiratory problems) do not necessarily apply to the same measure applied in a different context (e.g., 6-minute walk distance for patients with osteoarthritis of the knee). For this reason it is crucial to seek out studies that have evaluated a measure in a setting similar to your own. Criteria for evaluating a measure are presented in Chapter 10.

▶ Implementing the Best Measures for Your Practice

So far we have discussed prominent barriers and strategies to overcome the identified barriers when selecting outcome measures relevant to your practice. The next step is to devise an implementation strategy that ensures the continued successful use of these measures as essential decision-making aids. In this section we provide several ideas shared with us by physical therapists who have successfully implemented a comprehensive outcome assessment approach in their clinical settings.

- Involve your department's administrative staff when devising an implementation strategy. Although this comment may seem self-evident, leave this job to the experts. Your front office staff is key when it comes to ensuring that the appropriate outcome measures are available at the essential assessment time points. Let the administrative staff shape the implementation components for which they will be responsible.

- Consider time savers when administering self-report measures. Although previously, in the measure selection process, you have already considered the time it will take to administer a measure, having patients complete self-report measures prior to the actual therapist-patient interaction can further enhance efficiency. Examples of this include having patients complete a Web-based administration of the measure prior to coming to the clinic and having patients come in a few minutes early for their appointment and compete the self-report measure in the waiting room.

Use a single flowsheet to track all goals and outcome measures. The typical medical record is often organized chronologically. The initial assessment with the stated goals appears first, followed by progress notes. A limitation of using this format to track patient progress is the time required to locate and synthesize relevant information found at different places throughout a patient's chart. A second limitation is that it may not be obvious when a patient should be reassessed and for which outcome. A simple, yet extremely effective, strategy to overcome this limitation is to use a flowsheet that contains a patient's measurable goals, the outcomes and measures of interest, the reassessment dates, and when the goals have been met. Figure 9-1 displays an example of a flowsheet.

- Set up an efficient system to ensure the appropriate outcome measure resources (forms, stopwatch, tape measure, etc.) are available at the key reassessment time points. By placing the outcome measure tracking flowsheet in a common location in all patients' charts—such as fastened to the inside cover—the front office staff and physical therapist can quickly see when a reassessment is scheduled. In turn, the necessary arrangements can be made to ensure that the appropriate outcome measures and equipment are available when needed.

FUNCTIONAL GOAL AND OUTCOME FLOW-SHEET							
	DATE AND SCORE						
Date							
PAIN SCORE INTENSITY							
Patient-reported outcome measure score:							
Impairment measures to be followed:							
1.							
2.							
3.							
4.							
GOALS: (Enter date when goal is met)							
Measurable change goals							
1.							
2.							
3.							
4.							
Measurable change goals							
1.							
2.							
3.							
4.							

Figure 9-1 Functional Goal and Outcome Flowsheet. Courtesy of Jill Binkley.

Chapter Summary

- Choosing relevant outcome measures requires careful preparation.
- Being aware of potential barriers and implementing strategies to overcome these barriers can greatly enhance the chance of selecting the most appropriate outcome measures for your patients and practice.

- This chapter identifies potential barriers to the successful implementation of outcome measures and provides six barrier-busting steps to overcome them.

■ Reference List

1. Kay TM, Myers AM, Huijbregts MPJ. How far have we come since 1992? A comparative survey of physiotherapists' use of outcome measures. *Physiother Can* 2001;53:268–75, 81.

2. Stokes EK, O'Neill D. Use of outcome measures in physiotherapy practice in Ireland from 1998 to 2003 and comparison to Canadian trends. *Physiother Can* 2008;60:109–16.

3. Jette DU, Halbert J, Iverson C, Miceli E, Shah P. Use of standardized outcome measures in physical therapist practice: Perceptions and applications. *Phys Ther* 2009;89:125–35.

4. Copeland JM, Taylor WJ, Dean SG. Factors influencing the use of outcome measures for patients with low back pain: A survey of New Zealand physical therapists. *Phys Ther* 2008;88:1492–505.

5. Hazard RG, Haugh LD, Green PA, Jones PL. Chronic low back pain: The relationship between patient satisfaction and pain, impairment, and disability outcomes. *Spine* 1994;19:881–7.

6. Denis S, Shannon HS, Wessel J, Stratford P, Weller I. Association of low back pain, impairment, disability & work limitations in nurses. *J Occup Rehabil* 2007;17:213–26.

7. Mokkink LB, Terwee CB, Patrick DL, Alonso J, Stratford PW, Knol DL, et al. The COSMIN study reached international consensus on taxonomy, terminology, and definitions of measurement properties for health-related patient-reported outcomes. *J Clin Epidemiol* 2010;63:737–45.

8. Streiner DL, Norman GR. *Health Measurement Scales: A Practical Guide to Their Development and Use*, 4th ed. New York: Oxford University Press; 2008.

9. Messick S. Validity. In: Linn RL, editor. *Educational Measurement*, 3rd ed. Phoenix, AZ: ORYZ Press; 1993: p. 14.

Chapter 10

Finding and Critiquing Outcome Measures

■ *So far, we have discussed how information from outcome measures can be applied to guide clinical decisions. We have also introduced barriers to the successful clinical implementation of outcome measures, and have suggested six strategies for overcoming these barriers. In this chapter we describe an approach for finding relevant outcome measures and suggest criteria for evaluating them.*

▶ Finding Potential Outcome Measures of Interest for Your Unique Setting

We begin by describing an approach to locating potential outcome measures of interest and demonstrate an example of its implementation. The first step when seeking a relevant measure is to carefully construct a statement identifying your requirements for the measure. This statement is used to guide your search and subsequent decisions concerning the appropriateness of the candidate measures.

Once you have declared the measure's intended purpose and described your unique patients and clinical setting, administration and scoring considerations, and feasibility issues, the next step is to decide on the starting point for locating the measures. The starting point will vary depending on your knowledge of the breadth of outcome measures specific to your needs. Knowing the names of potential candidate measures is essential. If you are unaware of the names, finding a relevant measure may at first seem an overwhelming task. If this is the case, a number of options exist. Try searching Google Scholar or a database of outcome measures. Consult textbooks that list and describe outcome measures. Seek assistance from a colleague or your professional association. The following box lists examples of several databases and textbooks containing information on outcome measures.

Some Resources for Identifying Potential Outcome Measures

Websites
Google Scholar
http://scholar.google.ca/
Centre for Evidence Based Physiotherapy (CEBP), Maastricht
http://www.cebp.nl/?NODE=77
Patient-Reported Outcome and Quality of Life Instruments
  Database
http://www.proqolid.org/
Rehabilitation Measures Database
http://www.rehabmeasures.org/
StrokEngine Assess (specific to outcome measures specific to
  stroke)
http://www.medicine.mcgill.ca/strokengine-assess/
Transport Accident Commission of Australia
http://www.tac.vic.gov.au/jsp/content/NavigationController.do?a
  realD=22&tierID=1&navID=92ACB96A7F000001011DDD0
  421B6C947&navLink=null&pageID=942

Textbooks
McDowell I. *Measuring Health: A Guide to Rating Scales and
  Questionnaires,* 3rd ed. Oxford: Oxford University Press;
  2006.
Finch E, Brooks D, Stratford PW, Mayo NE. *Physical
  Rehabilitation Outcome Measures: A Guide to
  Enhanced Clinical Decision Making,* 2nd ed. Hamilton:
  BC Decker Inc; 2002.

Having identified one or more potential measures, the next step is to locate detailed information. Often, textbooks and databases do not include up-to-date information and one must turn to research studies. Accordingly, an effective and efficient literature search is required. Popular bibliographic databases and search engines include PubMed, Cumulative Index to Nursing and Allied Health Literature (CINAHL), Excerpta Medica (EMBASE), and Google Scholar.

- PubMed is a freely accessible service offered by the National Library of Medicine of the United States and it includes over 18 million citations from MEDLINE and other life science journals. (http://www.ncbi.nlm.nih.gov/sites/entrez)
- CINAHL is a comprehensive collection of nursing and allied health literature. CINAHL offers a free trial; however, for sustained use membership is required. (http://www.ebscohost.com/cinahl/)
- EMBASE contains biomedical and pharmacological citations. Like CINAHL, EMBASE offers a free trial; however, for ongoing use membership is required. (http://www.embase.com/)
- Google Scholar is a freely accessible Web search engine that indexes scholarly publications. (http://scholar.google.ca/)

Although similar search procedures are used with these databases, each has a unique syntax or method of constructing the search statement. Fortunately, tutorials are often available, and we recommend reviewing these tutorials before leaping into your own search.

▶ Overview of an Efficient Search Strategy

We define an efficient search strategy as one that yields the greatest number of relevant articles with the least amount of time and effort. Search terms play a key role in maximizing the efficiency and productivity of a search. Over the years we have identified three crucial components (set of terms) of a well-constructed search statement aimed at identifying outcome measure information. The first component is the name of the measure. Examples of outcome measure names include the Disabilities Arm Shoulder Hand measure (DASH), SF-36, 6-minute walk test, and grip strength. The second component is a list of the measurement terms related to the properties of interest. Although there are numerous possibilities, we have found those listed in Table 10–1 to be particularly effective. For example, if the goal is to focus on validity, the measurement component of the search statement would be as follows: (valid* OR psychometric OR clinimetric OR interpretab*). In the PubMed syntax, the asterisks (*) represent what is referred to as a "wild card." Wild cards allow the inclusion of all words with various combinations of letters following the asterisk (e.g., interpretable, interpretability).

The third component of the search statement is the condition or context of interest. Examples of conditions are stroke,

Table 10–1 Potential Terms to Be Included in the Measurement Component of the Search Statement

Reliability	Validity	Sensitivity to Change or Responsiveness
Reliability or reliab*	Validity (valid*)	Sensitivity
Standard error of measurement (SEM)	Psychometric Clinimetric Interpretability (interpretab*)	Responsiveness (responsiv*)
Intraclass correlation coefficient (ICC)		Receiver Operating Characteristic curve (ROC)
		Area under curve (AUC)
Bland		Clinically important change or difference (CIC, CID)
Psychometric Clinimetric		Minimal clinically important difference (MCID)
		Minimal clinically important change (MCIC)
		Minimal clinically important improvement (MCII)
		Minimal detectable change (MDC)
		Reliability change index (RCI)
		Change

osteoarthritis, chronic obstructive pulmonary disease, ankle sprain, and cerebral palsy.

In addition to these three essential components, adding a fourth element to the initial search is extremely useful. The goal of the fourth element is to identify systematic reviews for the outcome measure of interest. Systematic reviews represent a critical synthesis of previously published studies. Unlike a narrative review that parrots the findings of reported studies, a systematic review applies a specific methodology to locate, critique, and synthesize the relevant literature. Features of a well-conducted systematic review include a clearly stated question to be answered by the review, a comprehensive literature search with an explicit statement of the procedures used to identify the literature, a description of the methods used to obtain a reproducible abstraction of the information, a statement of the criteria and scoring methods used to critically appraise the relevant literature, and a synthesis of the findings. If a systematic review cannot be found or is outdated, the next step is to seek out and critically review recent primary research studies for the measure and context of interest.

▶ A Search Example

This example applies the concepts mentioned previously to identifying an outcome measure relevant for persons with low-back pain presenting to a physical therapy department. We present the steps from the perspective of a physical therapist seeking a measure for this purpose.

Step 1. *My statement of goals and constraints*
I wish to identify a standardized self-report measure of pain-related functional status that is sensitive to changes typically seen in outpatients presenting with acute, subacute, and chronic low-back pain and who are treated with interventions applied by physical therapists. Many patients with low-back pain seen in my clinic speak and read Spanish. Therefore, I wish to identify a standardized self-report measure of back-pain-related

functional status that has been validated in Spanish and English. Most patients should be able to complete the measure in under 5 minutes without assistance. I am willing to spend 30 seconds scoring the measure, provided computational aids (e.g., a calculator or computer) are not required. I am not willing to spend money purchasing a measure or equipment; however, I am willing to devote 3 hours of self-study time to learn how to use the measure.

Step 2.   *My starting point* I am not familiar with the names of potential measures. I went to Google Scholar first and typed in "low back outcome measure." Although this rather simple approach yielded over 1,600,000 hits, the first 4 proved extremely beneficial and included the following citation: Deyo RA, Battie M, Beurskens AJ, Bombardier C, Croft P, Koes B, et al. Outcome measures for low back pain research. A proposal for standardized use. *Spine* 1998;23:2003–13. The abstract for this study identified the Roland-Morris and Oswestry questionnaires as two recommended measures. As a matter of interest, 2 of the other first 4 citations included the Oswestry and Roland-Morris measures. Next, I went to the Centre for Evidence-based Physiotherapy (CEBP), Maastricht, website to find out more information. This site provided a copy of the Roland-Morris and its scoring criteria. Following this, I returned to Google and typed in Roland-Morris. In addition to providing references for scholarly peer-reviewed journal publications, this search also identified a website for the Roland-Morris measure (http://www.rmdq.org/). I learned that the Roland-Morris measure can be quickly scored without any computational aids. The Roland-Morris website also provided a list of languages for which the questionnaire is available. This list included Spanish.

Step 3.   *My literature search* Although a number of peer-reviewed citations were obtained from the Google Scholar search, I also conducted a PubMed literature search using the approach described previously. My initial search sought to identify systematic reviews of the Roland-Morris measure using the following search terms:

roland[tiab] AND (responsiv* OR sensitivity OR
psychometric OR clinimetric)
AND low+back AND systematic[tiab]

Applying this search statement yielded six citations, several of which appeared promising. Next, I repeated the search removing "systematic[tiab]." This search produced 126 hits. At this point I had two choices. I could review the titles and abstracts of the identified citations, or I could attempt to further refine my search terms in an attempt to reduce the number of citations. I chose the latter and included the word "change" in my search phrase:

roland[tiab] AND (responsiv* OR sensitivity OR
psychometric OR clinimetric)
AND low+back AND change

This search reduced the number of citations to 58. I elected to review the titles of these articles, and when a title appeared pertinent I also reviewed the abstract for relevance before deciding on whether to obtain a copy of the study. At this point, the Roland-Morris looked like a promising measure and I chose to review it in more detail.

Description of the Roland-Morris Measure

The Roland-Morris is a region-specific patient-reported outcome measure. It consists of 24 items. Each item is scored 1 if endorsed and 0 if left blank. Total Roland-Morris scores are obtained by summing the endorsed items. Thus, total scores can vary from 0 to 24, with higher scores representing greater levels of pain-related disability. It can be completed by most patients in 3 to 5 minutes and it can be scored in about 15 seconds without computational aids. Translated versions of this measure exist in over 30 languages and can be obtained free of charge at the following website: http://www.rmdq.org/. Given that the features of the Roland-Morris measure fulfill the feasibility requirements, the next step is to determine whether there exists sufficient information on the extent to which valid inferences can be drawn from Roland-Morris scores.

▶ Critiquing Outcome Measures

Determining the extent to which an outcome measure is proficient within a declared context is an ongoing process that cannot be captured in a single study. Support for a measure's ability is enhanced when the results from multiple well-conducted studies converge. Implicit in these statements is the notion that criteria exist for defining a well-conducted study or evaluating a body of information provided from multiple studies, but to our knowledge, there is no singularly agreed-upon set of criteria for evaluating the performance of an outcome measure within a declared context.

The criteria developed and presented by the Consensus-based Standards for the Selection of Health Measurement Instruments group (COSMIN) are perhaps the most comprehensive.[1–5] This group developed a critical appraisal tool (checklist) containing standards for evaluating the methodological quality of studies of patient-reported outcome measures. The checklist contains 10 sections and 107 items. The 10 sections are internal consistency (11 items), reliability (14 items), measurement error (11 items), content validity (5 items), structural validity (7 items), hypotheses testing (10 items), cross-cultural validity (15 items), criterion validity (7 items), responsiveness (18 items), and interpretability (9 items). A copy of this checklist and scoring criteria can be obtained at http://www.cosmin.nl/cosmin_1_0 .html. Although the COSMIN tool is an excellent resource for evaluating patient-reported outcome measures, some of its items are not applicable to performance measures. Also, because of its extensive nature it is time-consuming to complete and requires users to have a working knowledge of several advanced measurement concepts.

Rather than providing an exhaustive checklist for critically appraising outcome measures, we suggest six questions to consider when making a judgment concerning a measure. These questions are summarized in Table 10–2.

Table 10–2 Six Questions to Consider When Evaluating an Outcome Measure

Questions	Yes (Y), No (N), Can't tell (?)
1. Is the measure feasible to administer in your clinic?	
2. Has the measure been investigated on an unbiased sample?	
3. Has the measure been investigated on a sample of patients similar to patients seen in your practice?	
4. Was the methodology sufficiently rigorous to yield accurate estimates of the reliability, validity, and change coefficients?	
5. Is information available on (i) the confidence in a measured value? (ii) interpretation of a measured value? (iii) interpretation of a change value? (iv) a target value? (v) the anticipated change profile?	
6. Are the values associated with the five topics mentioned above of acceptable magnitude to guide clinical decision-making?	

Six Questions to Consider When Evaluating an Outcome Measure

1. *Is the measure feasible to administer in your clinic?*
   This question is straightforward. If you know it will not be practical to implement the measure in your setting, look for another measure.

2. *Has the measure been investigated on an unbiased sample?*
   We have learned previously that measurement properties are not properties of a measure, but rather how a measure performs in a specific context. The context includes the study setting and participant characteristics. If the spectrum of participants included in a study does not reflect a real-world situation, then the measurement properties obtained will have little meaning. Studies that include only patients with extreme change characteristics—that is, patients who remain unchanged or worsen and patients who change a great deal—will yield change coefficients that are different from those obtained had a real-world spectrum of patients been investigated. Random and consecutive sampling methods provide the best assurance of obtaining an unbiased sample. If you suspect an investigator has applied a biased sampling method, you can have little faith in the reported measurement properties.

3. *Has the measure been investigated on a sample of patients similar to patients seen in your practice?*
   This question differs from the previous one in that it is possible for an investigator to apply an unbiased sampling method and obtain a real-world spectrum of patients but the patients' characteristics are not similar to those seen in your setting. If this is the case, ask yourself, Are the patients taking part in the study so different from yours that the results are not likely to apply to your patients? If yes, you cannot be certain that the reported measurement properties will apply to your patients.

4. *Was the methodology sufficiently rigorous to yield accurate estimates of the reliability, validity, and change coefficients?* There are many subtleties involved in reviewing the methodological rigor of a measurement study. Here we highlight several key considerations for reliability, validity, and prognostic applications.

Test-retest reliability studies provide vital information concerning confidence in a measured value and when using minimal detectable change to guide decisions about true change. An important design consideration is the choice of reference standard used to identify patients who have not changed. Two approaches are widely used. One is to define a set interval between assessments over which patients are unlikely to change. The other is to apply a retrospective reference standard, such as a global rating of change, and have patients self-identify whether they believe they have changed or not. A disadvantage of the latter method is that the global rating of change and the outcome measure assessment are not independent because the patient completes both measures. This is likely to result in an overestimation of the reliability coefficient and an underestimation of the standard error of measurement and minimal detectable change. When reviewing the results, support for the assumption that patients have not truly changed can be found by comparing the means for the test and retest measurements. Although similar means do not ensure the stability of patients over the reassessment interval, a substantial difference in the means refutes the notion of stability. The final consideration is that the distribution of change scores, defined as the difference between test and retest values, must be consistent with a normal distribution. To ascertain whether this requirement holds, one looks for a formal test of normality. Frequently reported normality tests include the Shapiro-Wilk test and the Kolmogorov-Smirnov test. An alternate, albeit less rigorous, approach would be to make a judgment of normality based on a histogram or frequency distribution of change scores should either be available.

Investigators often apply correlational analysis when examining the validity of a measure's scores or change scores. Typically, an investigator hypothesizes that the correlation between measures believed to be assessing the same characteristic should correlate above some defined value (e.g., $r > 0.80$). In a situation such as this, it is essential that the analysis formally tests whether the obtained correlation exceeds the specified null r-value (i.e., 0.80 in this example). Too often, investigators base their decisions on the obtained point estimate and the p-value provided by the statistical software. Unfortunately, investigators often do not realize that the statistical software's output is reporting the p-value for the null hypothesis that $r = 0$, and not the null hypothesis that r is less than or equal to the specified null value. This concept also applies when evaluating other validity coefficients, such as the area under a receiver operating characteristic curve.

Identifying a high-quality reference standard is a methodological challenge when estimating a clinically important change. What makes this particularly challenging is that no gold standard exists for many important outcomes such as health or functional status. Often, investigators have applied a retrospective global rating of change that inquired about the amount of change as the reference standard. There are two methodological shortcomings here. First, and perhaps the most obvious, is that the investigators have asked about the amount of change rather than the importance of change. The second limitation is that the retrospective global rating of change is not independent of the measure's change scores. This lack of independence is likely to make the measure of interest appear better than it actually is. Although we are likely stuck with the retrospective global rating of change as one reference standard, we should seek out studies that apply different reference standards. Confidence in a threshold value of change is enhanced when the results of studies that applied different methodologies converge.

Our final methodological comment concerns investigations of the anticipated rate of change or prognosis. There are two key methodological considerations. One is that all patients are investigated from a common starting point for the disease or condition of interest. The second is that complete (or near complete) follow-up is achieved. If the former condition is not met, the apparent variation in patients' initial values and at the points in time patients reach their target value are likely to appear much greater than had all patients been initially assessed at a common point in time with respect to the condition of interest. In the latter case, patients not achieving complete follow-up may differ systematically from patients who do. This may result in either under- or overestimating the rate of change and target value.

In summary, if the methodological rigor of studies of a measure is severely compromised, look for another measure.

5. *Is information available on (a) the confidence in a measured value, (b) the interpretation of a measured value, (c) the interpretation of a change value, (d) a target value, and (e) the anticipated change profile?* The information referred to here is the substance of Chapters 4 to 8. If interpretive information is not available on these five topics, the measure may be of limited immediate use.

6. *Are the values associated with the topics identified in Point 5 of acceptable magnitude to guide clinical decision-making?* It is possible for an investigator to apply impeccable methodology and produce estimates of the relevant measurement properties and change coefficients, yet the values themselves indicate the measure is not performing at an acceptable level to be clinically useful. There is too much measurement error or uncertainty. If this is the case, look for another measure.

What We Found About the Roland-Morris Measure

Upon reviewing the studies identified from our literature search, we found the following. Many investigations of the Roland-Morris measure have applied an appropriate sampling method to patients receiving physical therapy.[6–10] Similar Roland-Morris mean values have been reported between test and retest, suggesting the measure is stable on truly unchanged patients.[11–13] Also, we found evidence that the distribution of difference values between test and retest values is consistent with a normal distribution.[11] Typical ICC estimates of test-retest reliability obtained in settings relevant to physical therapists are in the range of 0.79 to 0.88.[11,13–15] The SEM has been consistently estimated to be approximately 1.9 Roland-Morris points.[9,11,13,15] Applying a SEM of 1.9 produced a 90% confidence interval for a measured Roland-Morris value to be approximately ±3 points and a MDC_{90} of 4.4 points. One study applied diagnostic test methodology to estimate true change.[11] Using a retrospective global rating of change as the reference standard, this study estimated a true change threshold to be an improvement of 5 points. The reported area under the receiver operating characteristic (ROC) curve for this estimate was 0.88 (95% CI: 0.83, 0.92), and the sensitivity and specificity values were 0.63 (95% CI: 0.56, 0.70) and 0.98 (95% CI: 0.84, 1), respectively.

From these sensitivity and specificity values we computed the positive and negative predictive values, standardized to a pretest chance of improvement of 50%, to be 97% and 73%, respectively. Applying diagnostic test methodology, important improvement has been estimated to be approximately 5 points.[7,8,12] Reported areas under ROC curves vary from 0.68 to 0.93.[6–8,12] Combining typical sensitivity and specificity values of 0.72 and 0.82, respectively, with a pretest chance of improvement of 50% yields positive and negative predictive values of 80% and 75%, respectively.

We also found an estimate for a target value of recovery.[16] This study noted that a Roland-Morris score of less than or equal to 2 provided an accurate prediction of recovery.[16] Although this study did not report the sensitivity and specificity values for this threshold value, we were able to estimate them as 82% and 79% from a ROC curve figure shown in the paper. Assuming that the pretest chance of achieving recovery on reassessment is 50%, the positive and negative predictive values are approximately 80% and 81%, respectively. Because of the diverse and, in many instances, uncertain etiologies for low-back pain, limited information is currently available regarding the clinical course or change profile of patients.

Chapter Summary

In this chapter we described a search strategy for finding potential measures and proposed six questions to ask when deciding the likely usefulness of a measure in clinical practice. Taking the time and effort to locate the best measure for your needs can greatly reduce frustration and perhaps failure when implementing a new measure in your practice.

▪ Reference List

1. Mokkink LB, Terwee CB, Knol DL, Stratford PW, Alonso J, Patrick DL, et al. The COSMIN checklist for evaluating the methodological quality of studies on measurement properties: A clarification of its content. *BMC Med Res Methodol* 2010;10:22.

2. Mokkink LB, Terwee CB, Knol DL, Stratford PW, Alonso J, Patrick DL, et al. Protocol of the COSMIN study: COnsensus-based Standards for the selection of health Measurement INstruments. *BMC Med Res Methodol* 2006;6:2.

3. Mokkink LB, Terwee CB, Patrick DL, Alonso J, Stratford PW, Knol DL, et al. The COSMIN study reached international consensus on taxonomy, terminology, and definitions of measurement properties for health-related patient-reported outcomes. *J Clin Epidemiol* 2010;63:737–45.

4. Mokkink LB, Terwee CB, Patrick DL, Alonso J, Stratford PW, Knol DL, et al. The COSMIN checklist for assessing the methodological quality of studies on measurement properties of health status measurement instruments: An international Delphi study. *Qual Life Res* 2010;19:539–49.

5. Mokkink LB, Terwee CB, Gibbons E, Stratford PW, Alonso J, Patrick DL, et al. Inter-rater agreement and reliability of the COSMIN (COnsensus-based Standards for the selection of health status Measurement Instruments) checklist. *BMC Med Res Methodol* 2010;10:82.

6. Davidson M, Keating JL. A comparison of five low back disability questionnaires: Reliability and responsiveness. *Phys Ther* 2002;82:8–24.

7. Riddle DL, Stratford PW, Binkley JM. Sensitivity to change of the Roland-Morris Back Pain Questionnaire: Part 2. *Phys Ther* 1998;78: 1197–207.

8. Stratford PW, Binkley JM, Riddle DL, Guyatt GH. Sensitivity to change of the Roland-Morris Back Pain Questionnaire: Part 1. *Phys Ther* 1998;78: 1186–96.

9. Maughan EF, Lewis JS. Outcome measures in chronic low back pain. *European Spine Journal*: Official publication of the European Spine Society, the European Spinal Deformity Society, and the European Section of the Cervical Spine Research Society, 2010;19:1484–94.

10. Frost H, Lamb SE, Robertson S. A randomized controlled trial of exercise to improve mobility and function after elective knee arthroplasty. Feasibility, results and methodological difficulties. *Clin Rehabil* 2002;16:200–9.

11. Stratford PW, Riddle DL, Binkley JM. Assessing for changes in a patient's status: A review of current methods and a proposal for a new method of estimating true change. *Physiother Can* 2001;53:175–81.

12. Beurskens AJHM, de Vet HCW, Koke AJA. Responsiveness of functional status in low back pain: A comparison of different instruments. *Pain* 1996;65:71–6.

13. Ostelo RW, de Vet HC, Knol DL, van den Brandt PA. 24-item Roland-Morris Disability Questionnaire was preferred out of six functional status questionnaires for post-lumbar disc surgery. *J Clin Epidem* 2004;57: 268–76.

14. Riddle DL, Stratford PW. Roland-Morris scale reliability. *Phys Ther* 2002;82:512–5; author reply 5–7.

15. Demoulin C, Ostelo R, Knottnerus JA, Smeets RJ. What factors influence the measurement properties of the Roland-Morris disability questionnaire? *Eur J Pain* 2010;14:200–6.

16. Kamper SJ, Maher CG, Herbert RD, Hancock MJ, Hush JM, Smeets RJ. How little pain and disability do patients with low back pain have to experience to feel that they have recovered? *European Spine Journal*: Official publication of the European Spine Society, the European Spinal Deformity Society, and the European Section of the Cervical Spine Research Society, 2010;19:1495–501.

Chapter 11

Putting It All Together: Examples of the Application of Outcome Measures in Practice Settings

▪ *This chapter provides two case reports that illustrate the concepts introduced in this text. They are presented in a format that mirrors decisions encouraged in clinical practice. The first case involves a 63-year-old woman post total knee arthroplasty, and the second case considers a 20-month-old infant with cerebral palsy. We encourage you to read both cases, as they demonstrate somewhat different concepts.*

▪ Mrs. Janice Smith, *a 63-Year-Old Post Total Knee Replacement*

In this case we apply concepts introduced in Chapters 4 through 8 and 10.

Vignette

You are a physical therapist who has recently started work in a clinic that specializes in the rehabilitation of patients pre and post total joint arthroplasty. Mrs. Smith is the first patient you have seen in the clinic. She is an active woman with severe osteoarthritis of the right knee. Preoperatively, you assessed her 6-minute walk distance (6MWT) and obtained a value of

412 m. Mrs. Smith is now 2 weeks post total knee arthroplasty and her 6MWT distance is 232 m.

Questions

1. How confident can you be about Mrs. Smith's 6MWT distance of 232 m?

2. What is the interpretation of a 6MWT distance of 232 m?

3. How much change in Mrs. Smith's 6MWT distance is necessary to be reasonably certain that she has improved?

4a. When would the typical person with Mrs. Smith's 6MWT distance of approximately 232 m at 2 weeks post-arthroplasty be expected to improve by a detectable amount? Write a measurable goal.

4b. Suppose at 8 weeks post-arthroplasty Mrs. Smith had a 6MWT distance of 391 m. When would the typical person's 6MWT distance at 8 weeks post-arthroplasty be expected to improve by a detectable amount? Write a measurable goal.

5. What is Mrs. Smith's expected target 6-minute walk distance? How does distance compare to what the expected value would be for 63-year-old women in the population?

Approach to Questions and Responses

1. How confident can you be about Mrs. Smith's 6MWT distance of 232 m?

   To answer this question, we applied information reported in Chapters 4 and 10. The first step was to find studies reporting the reliability of the 6MWT for a similar patient group. Accordingly, we conducted a PubMed literature search using the following search themes: "measure AND measurement properties AND condition" format. We applied the following search term: ("6-min* walk" OR six-minute OR 6MW*) AND (reliab* OR SEM OR MDC OR test-retest) AND knee AND (osteoarthritis OR arthroplasty OR replacement).

Three articles were identified and we found the following one to be most relevant: Kennedy DM, Stratford PW, Wessel J, Gollish JD, Penney D. Assessing stability and change of four performance measures: A longitudinal study evaluating outcome following total hip and knee arthroplasty. *BMC Musculoskelet Disord* 2005;6:3. In this study Kennedy et al reported the relative reliability of the 6MWT to be 0.94 in a sample of patients with osteoarthritis of the knee awaiting total joint arthroplasty of the knee or hip. The standard error of measurement (SEM) was calculated to be 26.3 m. To obtain a 90% confidence interval for a patient's measured 6MWT distance, the SEM is multiplied by the z-value associated with the 90% confidence level (i.e., 1.65), and the product (26.3 × 1.65 = 43.4 m) is added and subtracted from the patient's measured value. For Mrs. Smith we interpret her 6MWT distance to be 232 ± 43.4 m.

2. What is the interpretation of a 6MWT distance in the range of 232 ± 43.4 m for a 63-year-old woman?

   To answer this question we applied the concepts presented in Chapter 5 to determine the 6MWT distance of a healthy age- and gender-matched person in the population. Our initial search used the following term: ("6-min* walk" OR six-minute OR 6MW*) AND ("reference") AND healthy.

This search produced 46 citations. We noticed that a number of these citations were specific to children. Accordingly, we modified our search terms as follows: ("6-min* walk" OR six-minute OR 6MW*) AND ("reference") AND healthy NOT children. This search produced 34 citations, several of which appeared promising. We reviewed the abstracts of these articles and identified the following citation by Casanova et al for review: Casanova C, Celli BR, Barria P, Casas A, Cote C, de Torres JP, et al. The 6-min walk distance in healthy subjects: Reference standards from seven countries. *The European Respiratory Journal*: Official journal of the European Society for Clinical Respiratory Physiology. 2011;37:150–6. This article suggested that a 6MWT distance of 580 m would be expected for a woman of approximately 63 years of age. Accordingly, we interpret Mrs. Smith's 6MWT distance of approximately 232 m to represent a substantial limitation in her ambulatory ability.

3. How much change in her 6MWT distance is necessary to be reasonably certain that Mrs. Smith has improved?

To answer this question we applied information discussed in Chapter 6 and began by conducting a literature search targeting change. Our search statement was as follows: ("6-min* walk" OR six-minute OR 6MW*) AND (MCID OR MCII OR MDC OR ROC OR sensitivity OR responsiv*) AND knee AND (osteoarthritis OR arthroplasty OR replacement).

Our search yielded 6 citations; however, only the article by Kennedy et al was specific to persons with end-stage osteoarthritis awaiting total knee or hip replacement. This study reported MDC_{90} to be 61 m. We did not locate a study that estimated true or important change using diagnostic test methodology or the percentile improvement methods. Applying the results from the study of Kennedy et al, we would need to see a change in Mrs. Smith's 6MWT distance of 61 m or more to be reasonably certain a true change has occurred.

4a. When would the typical person with Mrs. Smith's 6MWT distance of approximately 232 m at 2 weeks post-arthroplasty be expected to improve by a detectable amount? Write a measurable goal.

To answer this question we considered the concepts presented in Chapters 6 and 8. We applied the following search terms to locate potential studies that provide growth curves or change trajectories for persons post total knee arthroplasty: ("6-min* walk" OR six-minute OR 6MW*) AND (change OR growth OR trajectory OR curve OR percentiles OR prognos*) AND knee AND (arthroplasty OR replacement).

Our search produced 6 citations, however, only the following article provided change trajectories: Kennedy DM, Stratford PW, Riddle DL, Hanna SE, Gollish JD. Assessing recovery and establishing prognosis following total knee arthroplasty. *Phys Ther* 2008;88:22–32. The results from this study indicate that the change trajectory is influenced by a person's pre-arthroplasty 6MWT distance. In addition, the article by Kennedy et al provides an equation for deriving change trajectories for persons with different baseline 6MWT distances. Figure 11-1 displays

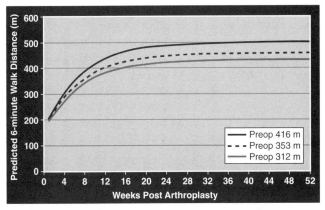

Figure 11-1 6MWT Change Trajectories by Three Different Pre-arthroplasty Distances for Females Post Total Knee Arthroplasty. Adapted from Kennedy DM, Stratford PW, Riddle DL, Hanna SE, Gollish JD. Assessing recovery and establishing prognosis following total knee arthroplasty. *Phys Ther* 2008;88:22–32. Reprinted with permission.

change trajectories for groups of persons with three different pre-arthroplasty 6MWT distances.

Applying Mrs. Smith's pre-arthroplasty 6MWT distance of 412 m to Figure 11-1, we would expect the typical person to be capable of walking approximately 240 m 2 weeks after arthroplasty. Considering Mrs. Smith's current 6MWT distance is 232 m (90% confidence interval ±43.4 m), we interpret Mrs. Smith's progress to be consistent with the typical female post-arthroplasty.

Two essential components of a measurable goal addressing change are the amount of change and the interval over which the change is expected to occur. The minimum amount of expected change would be set at the threshold value for detectable change. We learned previously that the threshold change value for the 6MWT is 61 m. The next step is to refer to the change trajectory curve and determine when the typical person 2 weeks post-arthroplasty who had a pre-arthroplasty 6MWT distance of 412 m would be expected to improve by

61 m. Examining Figure 11-1, we see that the person 2 weeks post-arthroplasty would be expected to improve 61 m in approximately 2 weeks. Thus, our measurable goal could be written as follows: To increase Mrs. Smith's 6MWT distance by 61 m in 2 weeks.

4b. Suppose at 8 weeks post-arthroplasty Mrs. Smith had a 6MWT distance of 391 m. When would the typical person with this walk distance at 8 weeks post-arthroplasty be expected to improve by a detectable amount? Write a measurable goal.

To answer this question we applied the same process as described above. Referring to Figure 11-1, we see that the rate of change has slowed down by 8 weeks post-arthroplasty and it would take the typical person approximately 4 weeks to improve 61 m. Accordingly, our measurable goal would be as follows: To increase Mrs. Smith's 6MWT distance by 61 m in 4 weeks.

5. What is Mrs. Smith's expected target 6-minute walk distance? How does distance compare to what the expected value would be for 63-year-old women in the population?

The answer to this question lies in the information provided in Chapter 7. We learned that persons with some conditions and characteristics would be expected to achieve a full recovery, and the target value for others will be less than that expected for the general population. The best evidence for a target value is based on condition- and person-specific values. For persons post-arthroplasty, we can apply information from trajectory curves, provided that the sample used was followed until a steady state was obtained. By steady state we mean that no further progress for the outcome of interest would occur. Referring to Figure 11-1, we see that Mrs. Smith would be expected to obtain a 6MWT distance of approximately 500 m. Even after accounting for measurement error, this distance is somewhat less than what would be expected for a healthy woman in the general population (approximately 580 m).

■ Sammy Scott, an Infant with Cerebral Palsy

In this case we apply concepts introduced in Chapters 4 through 8 and 10.

Vignette

You are a newly graduated physical therapist who has just started work in a pediatric clinic for infants with potential development problems. Your first patient is Sammy Scott, a 20-month-old infant with spastic diplegia. Sammy's family has recently moved into the community and he is being assessed for the first time. Sammy's parents have many questions; however, the one they are most concerned with is whether Sammy will eventually be able to walk.

Your clinic routinely applies the Gross Motor Functional Scale, 66-item version (GMFS-66) and the Gross Motor Function Classification System (GMFCS). The GMFM-66 is a criterion-referenced observational measure that was developed to assess children with cerebral palsy (CP).[1] The GMFCS is a five-level gross motor classification system that can be used to assist in estimating the expected change in motor function as a child becomes older.[2] You administer the GMFM-66 and obtain a score of 45.1 for Sammy.

Questions

1. How confident can you be about Sammy's GMFM-66 score of 45.1?
2. What is the interpretation of a GMFM-66 score of 45.1?
3. How much change in Sammy's GMFM-66 score is necessary to be reasonably certain that Sammy has improved an important amount?
4. When would the typical infant with Sammy's score be expected to improve an important amount?
5. What is Sammy's expected target GMFM-66 score? Is the typical child with this score likely to walk?

Approach to Questions and Responses

1. How confident can the therapist be about Sammy's GMFM-66 score of 45.1?

To answer this question we applied information reported in Chapters 4 and 10. The first step was to find studies reporting the reliability of the GMFM-66 for a similar patient group. Accordingly, we conducted a PubMed literature search applying the following search themes: "measure AND measurement properties AND condition." Our specific search terms were as follows: GMFM-66 AND (reliab* OR SEM OR MDC OR test-retest) AND (cerebral palsy OR CP).

This search produced 6 citations; however, the only apparent relevant article was in Chinese. Accordingly, we expanded by measurement terms as follows: GMFM-66 AND (reliab* OR SEM OR MDC OR test-retest OR sensitiv* OR responsiv* OR curve*) AND (cerebral palsy OR CP). This search yielded 11 articles with the following citation being most relevant: Wang HY, Yang YH. Evaluating the responsiveness of 2 versions of the Gross Motor Function Measure for Children with cerebral palsy. *Arch Phys Med Rehabil* 2006;87:51–56.

Although the primary goal of Wang's study was to compare the responsiveness of the GMFM-66 and GMFM-88, the authors did report the standard deviation of the difference score between two GMFM-66 measurements (2.6 points) for 11 children deemed not to have improved. We applied the following formula to their data:

$$SEM = \frac{\text{standard deviation of difference}}{\sqrt{2}}$$

and calculated the SEM to be 1.84 points. To obtain a 90% confidence interval (CI) for Sammy's GMFM-66 score, we multiplied the SEM by the z-value associated with a 90% CI (i.e., 1.65) and combined it with his obtained score as follows: 45.1 ± 1.65 × SEM. Thus, the 90% CI for Sammy's score is 42.1 to 48.1 GMFM-66 points. Accordingly, when forming an impression of Sammy's current functional level we consider his ability level to lie somewhere between 42.1 and 48.1 rather than exactly at 45.1.

2. What is the interpretation of a GMFM-66 score in the 42.1 to 48.1 range?

This question can be subdivided into three questions. To what extent does the GMFM-66 assess what it is intended to assess in the context of interest? What is the activity profile for a typical child with a GMFM-66 score in the 42.1 to 48.1 range? What GMFCS classification level is consistent with the activity profile of a typical child with a GMFM-66 score of 45.1? GMFCS levels are of interest because they provide prognostic information concerning a child's motor development.

To answer these questions we applied concepts introduced in Chapter 5. Once again, our first step was to locate studies that would clarify the interpretation of GMFM-66 scores and we applied the following search terms: GMFM-66 AND (IRT OR rasch OR understand* OR meaning OR scaling) AND (cerebral palsy OR CP).

This search yielded 8 citations and we found the following citation to be most relevant: Russell DJ, Avery LM, Rosenbaum PL, Raina PS, Walter SD, Palisano RJ. Improved scaling of the gross motor function measure for children with cerebral palsy: Evidence of reliability and validity. *Phys Ther* 2000;80:873–875. This article provided support for the validity of inferences drawn from GMFM-66 scores. Moreover, it included an item map that displays typical activity profiles for the spectrum of GMFM-66 scores. Referring to this item map, we determined that the typical child with a GMFM-66 score similar to Sammy's is able to crawl, pull himself to stand, and sit unassisted, occasionally using his hands for balance. These activity levels are consistent with a GMFCS Level II.

3. How much change in Sammy's GMFM-66 score is necessary to be reasonably certain that Sammy has improved an important amount?

To answer this question we applied information provided in Chapter 6 and began by conducting a literature search targeting change. Our search statement was as follows: GMFM-66 AND (MCID OR MCII OR MDC OR ROC OR sensitivity OR responsiv*) AND (cerebral palsy OR CP).

This search returned 6 citations of which the following study's findings were most relevant: Wang HY, Yang YH. Evaluating the responsiveness of 2 versions of the Gross Motor Function

Measure for Children with cerebral palsy. *Arch Phys Med Rehabil* 2006;87:51–56. Applying diagnostic test methodology, Wang et al reported an improvement to be 1.58 points or more (sensitivity 0.72, specificity 0.82) and a large (important) improvement to be 3.71 points or more (sensitivity 0.72, specificity 0.92).

Translating the sensitivity and specificity values reported by Wang et al into predictive values standardized to a pretest chance of improvement of 50% using the method shown in Chapter 6 yields the following:

	Positive Predictive Value	Negative Predictive Value
Improvement	80%	75%
Great (important) improvement	90%	77%

Our interpretation is that we can be reasonably certain (approximately 90%) that a child displaying an improvement greater than 3.71 GMFM-66 change points has truly improved an important amount.

4. When would the typical infant with Sammy's score at 20-months be expected to improve an important amount? *To answer this question we refer to concepts discussed in Chapters 6 and 8. Our first step is to seek out growth curves that display the expected change (development) over time in GMFM-66 scores for children similar to Sammy. We did this by applying the following search terms: GMFCS AND GMFM-66 AND (change OR growth OR trajectory OR curve OR percentiles OR prognos*) AND (cerebral palsy OR CP).* This search yielded 8 citations and the following study was most relevant: Hanna SE, Bartlett DJ, Rivard LM, Russell DJ. Reference curves for the Gross Motor Function Measure: Percentiles for clinical description and tracking over time among children with cerebral palsy. *Phys Ther* 2008;88:596–607.

Applying the growth curves (Fig. 11-2) reported by Hanna et al, we would expect the typical GMFCS Level II child assessed at 20 months to improve by 3.71 or more points in approximately 6 months. Accordingly, we scheduled Sammy's follow-up assessment to take place in 6-months time.

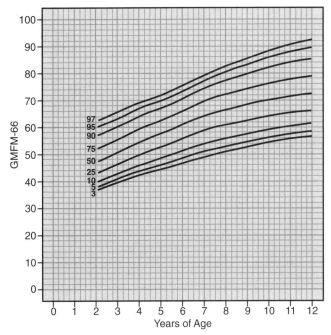

Figure 11-2 Gross Motor Function Classification System level II
Percentiles. (© 2008, SE Hanna, reprinted with permission.)

5. What is Sammy's expected target GMFM-66 score? Is the
typical child with this score likely to walk?
*To answer this question we applied information introduced
in Chapter 7 and again turned to the study of Hanna et al
used in Question 4. Their work shows (Fig. 11-2) that the
typical child with characteristics similar to Sammy (i.e.,
GMFCS Level II) will obtain a GMFM-66 score of
approximately 70.*
To answer the question posed by Sammy's parent, "Will Sammy
be able to walk?" we referred to the item map reported in the
publication by Russell et al and determined the functional
abilities of the typical child with a GMFM-66 score of 70 points.
In responding to Sammy's parents, we believe it is essential to
frame our answer in terms of a typical child with Sammy's

characteristics and current ability level, rather than Sammy specifically.

■ Reference List (Sammy Smith)

1. Russell DJ, Avery LM, Rosenbaum PL, Raina PS, Walter SD, Palisano RJ. Improved scaling of the gross motor function measure for children with cerebral palsy: Evidence of reliability and validity. *Phys The*r 2000;80: 873–85.

2. Palisano RJ, Hanna SE, Rosenbaum PL, Russell DJ, Walter SD, Wood EP, et al. Validation of a model of gross motor function for children with cerebral palsy. *Phys Ther* 2000; 80:974–85.

Index

Note: *f* denotes figure; *t*, table

A

Activity (ICF dimension), 13
  definition of, 15*t*
  examples of, 14*t*
  outcome measures of, 19–20, 20*t*, 22
  relationship between impairment and level of, 40
  subdomains of, 16*t*
Analysis of variance, 64
Anticipated problem, 29, 30, 31
Area under the curve (AUC), 77–78

B

Baseline and clinically important change, 97–99
Between-group difference, 96
Body functions and structures (ICF dimension), 13
  common outcomes of, 20*t*
  definition of, 15*t*
  examples of, 14*t*
  ICF subdomains of, 16*t*
  outcome measures of, 18–19, 22–23

C

Case reports
  63-year-old post total joint arthroplasty, 161–66, 165*f*
  infant with cerebral palsy, 167–72
Change. *See* Clinically important change; Prognosis
Change profile, 119–20, 120–22, 121*f*
Clinical course, growth curve model of, 120–22, 121*f*, 124–26
Clinical Examples
  growth curve and change profile, 121*f*, 123–24
    multiple studies, 125, 125*t*, 126*f*
  reassessment interval, 128, 129*t*
  reliability study, 55–56